T0183831

Lecture Notes in Computer Science 11075

Commenced Publication in 1973
Founding and Former Series Editors:
Gerhard Goos, Juris Hartmanis, and Jan van Leeuwen

More information about this series at http://www.springer.com/series/7412

Wenjia Bai · Gerard Sanroma
Guorong Wu · Brent C. Munsell
Yiqiang Zhan · Pierrick Coupé (Eds.)

Patch-Based Techniques in Medical Imaging

4th International Workshop, Patch-MI 2018
Held in Conjunction with MICCAI 2018
Granada, Spain, September 20, 2018
Proceedings

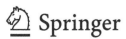 Springer

Editors
Wenjia Bai
Imperial College London
London, UK

Gerard Sanroma
German Center
  for Neurodegenerative Diseases
Bonn, Germany

Guorong Wu
University of North Carolina at Chapel Hill
Chapel Hill, NC, USA

Brent C. Munsell
College of Charleston
Charleston, SC, USA

Yiqiang Zhan
Shanghai Jiao Tong University
Shanghai, China

Pierrick Coupé
University of Bordeaux
Talence Cedex, France

ISSN 0302-9743   ISSN 1611-3349 (electronic)
Lecture Notes in Computer Science
ISBN 978-3-030-00499-6   ISBN 978-3-030-00500-9 (eBook)
https://doi.org/10.1007/978-3-030-00500-9

Library of Congress Control Number: 2018953883

LNCS Sublibrary: SL6 – Image Processing, Computer Vision, Pattern Recognition, and Graphics

This Springer imprint is published by the registered company Springer Nature Switzerland AG
The registered company address is: Gewerbestrasse 11, 6330 Cham, Switzerland

Preface

Patch-based techniques play an increasing role in the medical imaging field, with various applications in image segmentation, image de-noising, image super-resolution, super-pixel/voxel-based analysis, computer-aided diagnosis, image registration, abnormality detection, and image synthesis. Dictionaries of local image patches are increasingly being used in the context of segmentation and computer-aided diagnosis. Patch-based dictionaries are commonly used in conjunction with pattern recognition techniques to model complex anatomies in an accurate and easy way. The patch-level representation of image content is between the global image and localized voxel representations. This level of representation is shown to be successful in areas such as image processing (e.g., enhancement and de-noising) as well as image feature extraction and classification (e.g., convolution kernels and convolutional neural networks).

The aim of this workshop is to help advance scientific research within the broad field of patch-based processing in medical imaging. It focuses on major trends and challenges in this area, and it presents work aimed at identifying new cutting-edge techniques and their use in medical imaging. We hope that this workshop series will become a new platform for translating research from bench to bedside and for presenting original, high-quality submissions on innovative research and development in the analysis of medical image data using patch-based techniques.

Topics of interests include but are not limited to patch-based processing dedicated to:

- Image segmentation of anatomical structures or lesions (e.g., brain segmentation, cardiac segmentation, MS lesions detection, tumor segmentation)
- Image enhancement (e.g., de-noising or super-resolution dedicated to fMRI, DWI, MRI, or CT)
- Computer-aided prognostic and diagnostic (e.g., for lung cancer, prostate cancer, breast cancer, colon cancer, brain diseases, liver cancer, acute disease, chronic disease, osteoporosis)
- Mono and multimodal image registration
- Multi-modality fusion (e.g., MRI/PET, PET/CT, projection X-ray/CT, X-ray/ultrasound) for diagnosis, image analysis, and image-guided interventions
- Mono and multi modal image synthesis (e.g., synthesis of missing a modality in a database using an external library)
- Image retrieval (e.g., context-based retrieval, lesion similarity)
- Dynamic, functional, physiologic, and anatomic imaging
- Super-pixel/voxel-based analysis in medical images
- Sparse dictionary learning and sparse coding
- Analysis of 2D, 2D+t, 3D, 3D+t, 4D, and 4D+t data.

An academic objective of the workshop is to bring together researchers in medical imaging to discuss new techniques using patch-based approaches and their use in clinical decision support and large cohort studies. Another objective is to explore new paradigms of the design of biomedical image analysis systems that exploit the latest results in patch-based processing and exemplar-based methods. MICCAI-PatchMI 2018 featured a single-track workshop with keynote speakers, technical paper presentations, poster sessions, demonstrations of the state-of-the-art techniques, and concepts that are applied to analyzing medical images.

We received a total of 17 valid submissions. All papers underwent a rigorous double-blind review process by at least 2 members of the Program Committee composed of well-known experts in the field. The selection of the papers was based on significance of results, technical merit, relevance, and clarity of presentation. Based on the reviewing scores and comments, 15 papers were accepted for presentation at the workshop and chosen to be included in the present proceedings.

August 2018

W. Bai
G. Sanroma
G. Wu
Brent C. Munsell
Y. Zhan
P. Coupé

Organization

Program Committee

Charles Kervrann	Inria Rennes - Bretagne Atlantique, France
Daoqiang Zhang	Nanjing University of Aeronautics and Astronautics, China
Dinggang Shen	UNC Chapel Hill, USA
Francois Rousseau	IMT Atlantique, France
Gang Li	UNC Chapel Hill, USA
Guoyan Zheng	University of Bern, Switzerland
Hongzhi Wang	IBM Almaden Research Center, USA
Islem Rekik	University of Dundee, UK
Jean-Francois Mangin	I2BM, France
Jose Manjon	ITACA institute, Universidad Politècnica de Valencia, Spain
Junzhou Huang	University of Texas at Arlington, USA
Jussi Tohka	Universidad Carlos III de Madrid, Spain
Karim Lekadir	Universitat Pompeu Fabra, Spain
Li Shen	University of Pennsylvania, USA
Li Wang	UNC Chapel Hill, USA
Martin Styner	UNC Chapel Hill, USA
Olivier Colliot	UPMC, France
Olivier Commowick	Inria, France
Qian Wang	Shanghai Jiao Tong University, China
Rolf Heckemann	Sahlgrenska University Hospital, Sweden
Sailesh Conjeti	German Center of Neurodegenerative Diseases, Germany
Simon Eskildsen	Center of Functionally Integrative Neuroscience, Denmark
Weidong Cai	University of Sydney, Australia
Yong Fan	University of Pennsylvania, USA

Contents

Brain Image Analysis

Retinal Image Analysis

Image Denoising

Learning Real Noise for Ultra-Low Dose Lung CT Denoising

Michael Green[1], Edith M. Marom[2], Eli Konen[2], Nahum Kiryati[1],
and Arnaldo Mayer[2(✉)]

[1] Department of Electrical Engineering, Tel-Aviv University, Tel Aviv, Israel
greenl@mail.tau.ac.il, nk@eng.tau.ac.il
[2] Diagnostic Imaging, Sheba Medical Center, Affiliated to the Sackler School
of Medicine, Tel-Aviv University, Tel Aviv, Israel
{edith.marom, eli.konen,
arnaldo.mayer}@sheba.health.gov.il

Abstract. Neural image denoising is a promising approach for quality enhancement of ultra-low dose (ULD) CT scans after image reconstruction. The availability of high-quality training data is instrumental to its success. Still, synthetic noise is generally used to simulate the ULD scans required for network training in conjunction with corresponding normal dose scans. This reductive approach may be practical to implement but ignores any departure of the real noise from the assumed model. In this paper, we demonstrate the training of denoising neural networks with real noise. For this purpose, a special training set is created from a pair of ULD and normal-dose scans acquired on each subject. Accurate deformable registration is computed to ensure the required pixel-wise overlay between corresponding ULD and normal-dose patches. To our knowledge, it is the first time real CT noise is used for the training of denoising neural networks. The benefits of the proposed approach in comparison to synthetic noise training are demonstrated both qualitatively and quantitatively for several state-of-the art denoising neural networks. The obtained results prove the feasibility and applicability of real noise learning as a way to improve neural denoising of ULD lung CT.

1 Introduction

Neural image denoising and its application to low-dose CT scans has become a dynamic field of research [1–8]. In [1], the patches sequentially extracted from the input slice by a 2-D sliding window are processed by a multi-layer perceptron and directly replaced by the denoised output patch. The denoised image is obtained by spatial averaging of the overlapping output patches. A fully-connected neural network is trained in [2] to denoise coronary CT angiography patches. The denoised image is generated by a locally-consistent non-local-means algorithm [9] applied to the denoised patches.

In [3], a convolutional neural network (CNN) is proposed for denoising. The CNN layers are purely convolutional, each one being followed by batch-normalization [10] and a (rectified linear unit) ReLU non-linearity. To improve denoising performance, the

© Springer Nature Switzerland AG 2018
W. Bai et al. (Eds.): Patch-MI 2018, LNCS 11075, pp. 3–11, 2018.
https://doi.org/10.1007/978-3-030-00500-9_1

residual between ground-truth (GT) and input, thus representing a noise image, is learned by the network instead of the habitual mapping between noisy input and GT image.

In [4], a denoised instance of the input image is first computed by the classical BM3D algorithm [11]. Next, similar image patches from the denoised instance, are stacked together into blocks with noisy image patches extracted at the same position. The blocks are subsequently denoised by the network proposed in [3] and the output image is obtained by aggregation of the denoised patches.

In [5], a 3-layers fully CNN (FCNN) is trained on pairs of corresponding clean and noisy CT patches. The noisy images, from which the training patches are extracted, are generated by Poisson noise addition to the clean images in the sinogram domain. L_2 distance metric is used for network loss computation. Leveraging the FCNN architecture, training on image patches allows for direct denoising of full size images.

A perceptual loss was proposed in [6] as an improvement to the commonly used L_2 loss between denoised and original clean images. The perceptual loss is computed in a high-dimensional feature space generated by the well-known VGG network [12]. The proposed CNN is trained to minimize the L_2 loss between the VGG features extracted from the denoised image and the same extracted from the GT clean image. In [7], a residual encoder-decoder architecture is proposed with skip connections. The encoding layers (convolutions) extract the image features, while the decoding layers successively reconstruct the denoised image from the extracted features (deconvolutions). Generative adversarial networks (GAN) [13] have also been proposed for low dose CT denoising in combination with a sharpness detection network to avoid oversmoothing of the output [8].

While previous works have proposed a variety of network architectures, they all share a basic limitation dictated by convenience: the networks are trained on synthetic data obtained by artificial addition of parametric noise, usually assumed to be Poisson-distributed, in the sinogram domain. Consequently, any departure from the assumed noise model is ignored. In this work, we propose the training of denoising networks with a dataset built on real ultra-low dose/normal-dose pairs of scans, acquired for each patient. The proposed approach allows, for the first time to our knowledge, the learning of real ultra-low dose (ULD) CT noise by denoising neural networks. The remainder of this paper is organized as follows: The construction of the real noise dataset is described in Sect. 2 and validated, both qualitatively and quantitatively, in Sect. 3. A discussion concludes the paper in Sect. 4.

2   Methods

A dataset of 20 cases was created by scanning each subject twice, once at normal dose and once at ULD. The normal-dose scan was acquired at 120 kVp under adaptive tube current modulation. The ULD scan was acquired at 120 kVp at a constant tube current of 10 or 20 mA for subjects with a body mass index (BMI) below or above 29, respectively. Prior written consent was obtained for each patient as required in the IRB authorization released by our institution. The cases consisted of adult subjects, over 18 years old for men, and 50 for women to avoid risks of undetected pregnancy.

The subjects were recruited among patients referred to a standard chest CT, with or without contrast media. The reduction in radiation dose (R) between normal and ULD scans is given by (Eq. 1):

$$R = 100 \cdot \left(1 - \frac{DLP_{ULD}}{DLP_{normal}}\right) \tag{1}$$

where DLP_{ULD}, and DLP_{normal} are the dose-length-product of the ULD and normal-dose scans, respectively. The average R across the dataset was about 94%. The dose report for a sample subject is shown in Fig. 1 with (green) $DLP_{normal} = 317.4\,\text{mGy.cm}$ and (red) $DLP_{ULD} = 13.58\,\text{mGy.cm}$, corresponding to R = 96%. Consequently, the additional radiation dose incurred by the patient undergoing the two scans is merely of 4%, keeping the overall radiation exposure (total exam DLP) at an acceptable level for a lung CT scan. The scans are performed at full inspiration under breath-hold. Since the total scan time may be too long for a single breath-hold, each scan is acquired under a separate one. However, as lung inflation is not exactly the same in both scans, a deformable registration step is required to ensure accurate pixel-wise overlay between the scans, so that pairs of corresponding normal-dose and ULD patches can be extracted to train the neural networks.

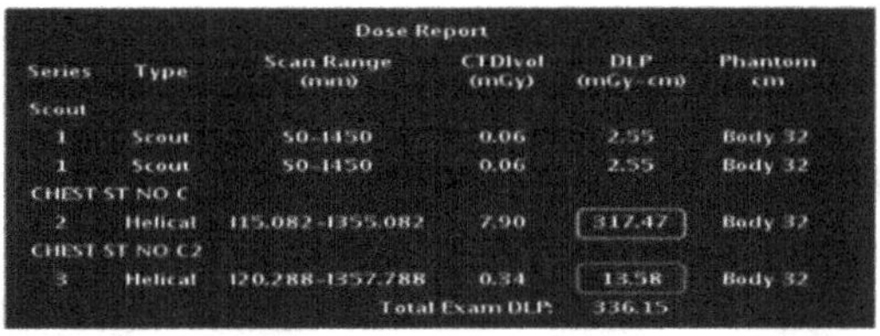

Dose Report

Series	Type	Scan Range (mm)	CTDIvol (mGy)	DLP (mGy-cm)	Phantom cm
Scout					
1	Scout	50-1450	0.06	2.55	Body 32
1	Scout	50-1450	0.06	2.55	Body 32
CHEST ST NO C					
2	Helical	115.082-1355.082	7.90	317.47	Body 32
CHEST ST NO C2					
3	Helical	120.288-1357.788	0.34	13.58	Body 32
			Total Exam DLP:	336.15	

Fig. 1. The dose report for a sample subject scanned twice: once at normal dose (series 2) and once at ULD (series 3). The respective DLPs are $DLP_{normal} = 317.4\,\text{mGy.cm}$ (green) and $DLP_{ULD} = 13.58\,\text{mGy.cm}$ (red), corresponding to R = 96%. (Color figure online)

The registration process involves two images: a fixed image (I_F) and a moving image (I_M). It recovers a spatial transformation $T(x) = x + u(x)$ such that $I_M(T(x))$ is spatially aligned to $I_F(x)$. To compute $T(x)$, the formulation of the Elastix package [14] was used with a third order b-spline parametrization. Minimization was performed for the cost function given by (Eq. 2):

$$C(T; I_F, I_M) = -S(T; I_F, I_M) + \gamma P(T) \tag{2}$$

where, S is a similarity function computed between I_F and $I_M(T(x))$ and P is a regularization function that constrains $T(x)$. *Mutual information* was chosen as function S, and *bending energy* as function P [14]. The γ parameter balances between similarity and regularity in the cost function. To compensate for small changes in patient position and orientation, a 3-D rigid transform (6 degrees of freedom) was first computed between the ULD and the normal-dose scans, before the deformable step. The parameter values for both registration steps were chosen as in [15]. The normal-dose scan was taken as reference image (I_F) for all the registration tasks. A sample case slice is shown in Fig. 2. The ULD image (a) is shown alongside the normal-dose (b) and co-registered ULD (T-ULD) (c) images. Highlighted ROIs (red, green, blue) are zoomed-in in (d): ULD (left column), normal-dose (middle) and T-ULD (right). The ULD ROIs (left) are clearly misaligned with the normal-dose ones (middle), while the latter are well aligned with the T-ULD ROIs. Before using the pairs of aligned patches to train neural networks, we perform a patch selection step in order to remove pairs with insufficient registration accuracy from the generated training set. We define the selected patch dataset D as (Eq. 3):

$$D = \{(p_i, q_i), SIM(p_i, q_i) > T_{SIM}\} \tag{3}$$

Where, p_i and q_i are normal-dose and T-ULD patch pairs, respectively, SIM is a similarity measure and T_{SIM} is a threshold. We used the structural similarity index (SSIM) [16] as the similarity measure and set empirically T_{SIM} to be 0.4. The underlying idea being that improved alignment accuracy will result in increased content similarity between the compared patches, leading to higher SSIM values. After selection, the resulting real-noise database contained about 700,000 patch pairs of size 45×45 pixels.

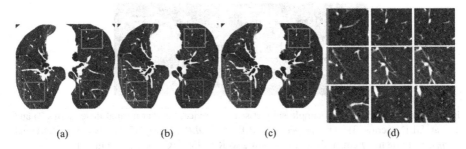

| (a) | (b) | (c) | (d) |

Fig. 2. Sample case slice: (a) ULD image; (b) normal-dose image; (c) co-registered ULD (T-ULD). (d) Zoom-in ROIs (red, green, yellow): ULD (left column), normal-dose (middle) and T-ULD (right). The ULD ROIs (left) are clearly misaligned with the normal-dose ones (middle), while the latter are well aligned with the T-ULD ROIs. (Color figure online)

3   Experiments

For the validation of the proposed approach, four state-of-the-art denoising CNN were implemented: LD-CNN [5], DnCNN [3], RED-CNN [7] and CNN-VGG [6]. Each architecture was trained in two different version: a first using the real-noise database, and a second using synthetic noise. The synthetic noise database was created using the ASTRA toolbox [17] by adding Poisson noise with $I_0 = 22 \times 10^4$ to the computed sinogram of each normal-dose image in order to simulate $R \sim 90\%$ [2].

A 5-folds cross-validation scheme was adopted. In each fold, 4 cases were used for testing and all the remaining, for training. In total, 40 different networks were created (5 folds × 4 architectures × 2 training sets). The quantitative comparison was performed between denoised T-ULD and normal-dose scans for SSIM and PSNR scores. Here again, to avoid affecting the denoising scores by registration inaccuracies, SSIM and PSNR were only computed at locations where (1) was satisfied. Note that the SSIM computed in (1) for patch selection is between normal-dose and T-ULD, whereas the SSIM of the validation is between denoised T-ULD and normal-dose. In Fig. 3, quantitative comparison of the PSNR (a–d) and SSIM (e–h) for the LD-CNN, DnCNN, RED-CNN and CNN-VGG networks is shown for each fold, following real (blue) and synthetic (red) noise training. The networks trained with real-noise, outperformed the SSIM (e–h) of their synthetic noise counterpart for all the folds and architectures. For PSNR (a–d), the same situation is observed, except for the third fold, in which CNN-VGG was the only network with higher PSNR for real-noise training. Also, it is interesting to note that although LD-CNN has a simple architecture, consisting of only three convolutional layers, it generated the best PSNR and SSIM scores in most of the cases. A possible reason may be that wider and shallow networks are better in capturing pixel-distribution features [18], a property which is critical in the case of real noise learning. Denoising results for a sample slice are shown in Fig. 4. The highlighted ROIs (red, green, yellow) in the ULD (a) and normal-dose images (b) are denoised and zoomed-in (c–f) by DnCNN (c), LD-CNN (d), RED-CNN (e) and CNN-VGG (f) for real (left columns) and synthetic (right columns) noise training. The results obtained for real-noise training appear sharper, with more fine details visible in comparison to the synthetic training results, which exhibit some over-smoothing. This is further verified by computing the overall image sharpness from the approximate sharpness map, $S_3(x)$, defined in [19] by (Eq. 4):

$$S_3(x) = \sqrt{S_1(x) \times S_2(x)} \qquad (4)$$

Where, $S_1(x)$ is a spectral-based sharpness map and $S_2(x)$ is a spatial based sharpness map. The overall image sharpness is given by the average of the top 1% values in $S_3(x)$ and is denoted by S_3 [19]. The average S_3 index computed on the denoised images for all the networks trained with real-noise (blue) and synthetic-noise (red) are shown in Fig. 5 for the 5 folds. In all, but one, fold of a single algorithm (CNN-VGG), the overall sharpness index was better for real-noise training than for synthetic, confirming the visual impression of Fig. 4.

In a last experiment, the local contrast of a tiny 2.5 mm lung nodule was compared after denoising with real and synthetic noise training. Figure 6 shows the ROI containing the nodule (a, top) zoomed-in after denoising (red arrow) by the four state-of-the-art CNNs (b–e). The nodule appears with stronger contrast for real-noise training (top row images) than for synthetic noise (bottom row images). This is further confirmed in Table 1, by the Michelson contrast, *MC*, [20] which computes the normalized difference between maximal and minimal intensities measured and averaged along radial profiles (green lines, (a)-bottom) of the nodule.

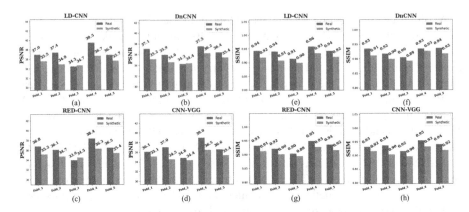

Fig. 3. Quantitative comparison of denoising results obtained by networks trained with real (blue) and synthetic (red) noise. The PSNR (a–d) and SSIM (e–h) scores are given for LD-CNN, DnCNN, RED-CNN and CNN-VGG, respectively. (Color figure online)

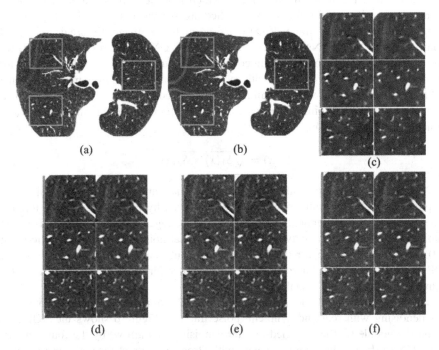

Fig. 4. A sample result slice. The highlighted ROIs (red, green, yellow) in the ULD (a) and normal-dose images (b) are denoised and zoomed-in (c–f) by DnCNN (c), LD-CNN (d), RED-CNN (e) and CNN-VGG (f) for real (left columns) and synthetic (right columns) noise training. The reader is encouraged to zoom in for a better assessment of sharpness. (Color figure online)

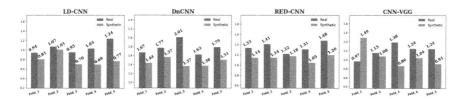

Fig. 5. The average S_3 values [19] of the denoising results obtained by networks trained with real (blue) and synthetic (red) noise. (Color figure online)

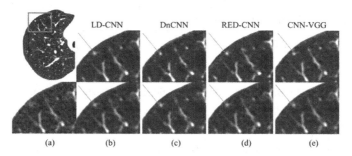

Fig. 6. Tiny lung nodule (a, top) in red ROI zoomed-in after denoising (red arrow) by the four state-of-the-art CNNs (b–e). The nodule appears with stronger contrast for real-noise training (top row images) than for synthetic noise (bottom row images). The Michelson contrast is computed along the green sampling lines (a, bottom) on the nodule. (Color figure online)

Table 1. The average Michelson contrast [20] around the nodule

Noise	LD-CNN	DnCNN	RED-CNN	CNN-VGG
Real	0.241	0.341	0.332	0.257
Synthetic	0.206	0.225	0.194	0.199

4 Conclusions

In this paper, the learning of real noise was proposed for neural network denoising of ULD lung CT. While synthetic noise has been widely used in prior works, it is the first time, to our knowledge, that real CT noise, extracted from real pairs of co-registered ULD and normal-dose scans, is used for training denoising neural networks. In particular, the proposed combination of deformable registration and double scanning enables the computation of quantitative denoising scores in real denoising tasks whereas these were only computed for synthetic noise in previous works. The benefits of the proposed approach were demonstrated on four state-of-the-art neural denoising architectures. Beside the improvement in PSNR and SSIM, a substantial improvement in image sharpness was observed for the images denoised using real-noise trained networks. Local contrast improvement was also demonstrated for a tiny lung nodule following denoising by the proposed approach. The obtained results suggest that the proposed approach is a promising way to improve neural denoising of ULD lung CT scans.

References

1. Burger, H.C., Schuler, C.J., Harmeling, S.: Image denoising: can plain neural networks compete with BM3D? In: IEEE Conference on Computer Vision and Pattern Recognition (CVPR) (2012)
2. Green, M., Marom, E.M., Kiryati, N., Konen, E., Mayer, A.: A neural regression framework for low-dose Coronary CT Angiography (CCTA) denoising. In: Wu, G., Munsell, B.C., Zhan, Y., Bai, W., Sanroma, G., Coupé, P. (eds.) Patch-MI 2017. LNCS, vol. 10530, pp. 102–110. Springer, Cham (2017). https://doi.org/10.1007/978-3-319-67434-6_12
3. Zhang, K., Zuo, W., Chen, Y., Meng, D., Zhang, L.: Beyond a gaussian denoiser: residual learning of deep CNN for image denoising. IEEE Trans. Image Process. **26**, 3142–3155 (2017)
4. Ahn, B., Cho, N.I.: Block-matching convolutional neural network for image denoising. arXiv preprint arXiv:1704.00524 (2017)
5. Chen, H., et al.: Low-dose CT via convolutional neural network. Biomed. Opt. Express **8**(2), 679–694 (2017)
6. Yang, Q., Yan, P., Kalra, M.K., Wang, G.: CT image denoising with perceptive deep neural networks. arXiv preprint arXiv:1702.07019 (2017)
7. Chen, H., et al.: Low-dose CT with a residual encoder-decoder convolutional neural network (RED-CNN). arXiv preprint arXiv:1702.00288 (2017)
8. Yi, X., Babyn, P.: Sharpness-aware low dose CT denoising using conditional generative adversarial network. arXiv preprint arXiv:1708.06453 (2017)
9. Green, M., Marom, E.M., Kiryati, N., Konen, E., Mayer, A.: Efficient low-dose CT denoising by locally-consistent non-local means (LC-NLM). In: Ourselin, S., Joskowicz, L., Sabuncu, M.R., Unal, G., Wells, W. (eds.) MICCAI 2016. LNCS, vol. 9902, pp. 423–431. Springer, Cham (2016). https://doi.org/10.1007/978-3-319-46726-9_49
10. Ioffe, S., Szegedy, C.: Batch normalization: accelerating deep network training by reducing internal covariate shift. In: International Conference on Machine Learning (2015)
11. Dabov, K., Foi, A., Katkovnik, V., Egiazarian, K.: Image denoising by sparse 3-D transform-domain collaborative filtering. IEEE Trans. Image Process. **16**(8), 2080–2095 (2007)
12. Simonyan, K., Zisserman, A.: Very deep convolutional networks for large-scale image recognition. arXiv preprint arXiv:1409.1556 (2014)
13. Goodfellow, I., et al.: Generative adversarial nets. In: Advances in Neural Information Processing Systems (2014)
14. Klein, S., Staring, M., Murphy, K., Viergever, M.A., Pluim, J.P.: Elastix: a toolbox for intensity-based medical image registration. IEEE Trans. Med. Imaging **29**(1), 196–205 (2010)
15. Sokooti, H., Saygili, G., Glocker, B., Lelieveldt, B.P.F., Staring, M.: Accuracy estimation for medical image registration using regression forests. In: Ourselin, S., Joskowicz, L., Sabuncu, M.R., Unal, G., Wells, W. (eds.) MICCAI 2016. LNCS, vol. 9902, pp. 107–115. Springer, Cham (2016). https://doi.org/10.1007/978-3-319-46726-9_13
16. Wang, Z., Bovik, A.C., Sheikh, H.R., Simoncelli, E.P.: Image quality assessment: from error visibility to structural similarity. IEEE Trans. Image Process. **13**(4), 600–612 (2004)

17. van Aarle, W., et al.: Fast and flexible X-ray tomography using the ASTRA toolbox. Opt. Express **24**(22), 25129–25147 (2016)

18. Liu, P., Fang, R.: Wide inference network for image denoising. arXiv preprint arXiv:1707. 05414 (2017)

19. Vu, C.T., Phan, T.D., Chandler, D.M.: S3: a spectral and spatial measure of local perceived sharpness in natural images. IEEE Trans. Image Process. **21**(3), 934–945 (2012)

20. Michelson, A.A.: Studies in Optics. Courier Corporation (1995)

MRI Denoising Using Deep Learning

José V. Manjón[1(✉)] and Pierrick Coupe[2,3]

[1] Instituto de Aplicaciones de las Tecnologías de la Información y de las
Comunicaciones Avanzadas (ITACA), Universitat Politècnica de València,
Camino de Vera s/n, 46022 Valencia, Spain
jmanjon@fis.upv.es
[2] Univ. Bordeaux, LaBRI, UMR 5800, PICTURA, 33400 Talence, France
[3] CNRS, LaBRI, UMR 5800, PICTURA, 33400 Talence, France

Abstract. MRI denoising is a classical preprocessing step which aims at
reducing the noise naturally present in MR images. In this paper, we present a
new method for MRI denoising that combines recent advances in deep learning
with classical approaches for noise reduction. Specifically, the proposed method
follows a two-stage strategy. The first stage is based on an overcomplete patch-
based convolutional neural network that blindly removes the noise without
estimation of local noise level present in the images. The second stage uses this
filtered image as a guide image within a rotationally invariant non-local means
filter. The proposed approach has been compared with related state-of-the-art
methods and showed competitive results in all the studied cases.

1 Introduction

Magnetic resonance image (MRI) denoising is key preprocessing step in many image
processing and analysis tasks. There is a large amount of papers related to this topic [1].
Most of denoising methods can be classified on those that use the intrinsic pattern
redundancy of the images and those exploiting their sparseness properties.

On the first class, the well-known non-local means (NLM) filter [2] is maybe the
most representative method. The bibliography related to extensions of this method is
quite extensive [3–5]. On the other hand, sparseness-based methods try to reduce the
noise by assuming that most of the signal can be sparsely represented using few basis
signals (using fixed basis like in FFT or DCT [6] or data dependent basis using for
example PCA [7]).

Recently, deep learning methods have also proposed to denoise MR images by
training different architectures with pairs of noisy and noise-free input-outputs. Such
methods try to infer the clean image from the noisy input. The main benefit of these
techniques is that after training, the denoising can be applied extremely fast (on GPUs).
One of the first deep learning methods for denoising was proposed by Gondara [8]
using convolutional denoising autoencoders though a bottleneck strategy to denoise 2D
images. Benou et al. [9] proposed a spatio-temporal denoising method using restricted
Boltzman machines. More recently, Jiang et al. [10] proposed a specific Rician noise
filter using a slice-wise convolutional neural network.

© Crown Copyright is asserted by the Australian Government 2018
W. Bai et al. (Eds.): Patch-MI 2018, LNCS 11075, pp. 12–19, 2018.
https://doi.org/10.1007/978-3-030-00500-9_2

In this paper, we present a novel denoising approach based on the application of a 3D Convolutional Neural Network using an overcomplete patch-based sliding window scheme. The resulting filtered image is used as a guide image to accurately estimate the voxel similarities within a rotationally invariant NLM (RI-NLM) strategy as done in Manjón et al. [7].

2   Materials and Methods

2.1   Image Data

Training Dataset: To train a supervised neural network a ground truth is needed to teach the network how the desired output looks like. Unfortunately, zero noise images do not exist and the only two options are to simulate noise free images or to work with a low-noise image resulted from the averaging of multiple acquired images and to consider it as a bronze standard. The first option has indeed images with zero noise but at the expense of a simpler and less realistic anatomy. The second is anatomically more complete but zeros noise condition is not met. In this paper, we have used both approaches.

MNI Synthetic Dataset: We used 20 simulated T1 brain MRIs from the MNI brain simulator. To train the network several levels of stationary Gaussian noise (1% to 9% of maximum intensity) were added to generate the training data.

IXI Dataset: Since to acquisition of several MRIs is a costly process we used as a surrogate denoised images from the IXI dataset. Specifically, we randomly selected 30 T1 MRIs from this dataset and we denoised them using the PRI-NL-PCA method [7] which is a state-of the-art-method. Denoised images had virtually almost zero noise and the anatomy was minimally affected by the application of the filter as can be checked in the residual image obtained by subtracting the noisy and denoised image. Again, to train the network several levels of stationary Gaussian noise were added to generate the training data (1% to 9% of maximum intensity).

Test Dataset: To be able to quantitatively compare the proposed method with previous methods, we used the well-known Brainweb 3D T1-weighted MRI phantom [11] as test dataset. This synthetic dataset has a size of $181 \times 217 \times 181$ voxels (voxel resolution = 1 mm^3) and was corrupted with different levels of stationary Gaussian and Rician noise (1% to 9% of maximum intensity). Rician noise was generated by adding Gaussian noise to real and imaginary parts and then computing the magnitude image.

2.2   Preprocessing

Classic preprocessing in deep learning consist of center the images by subtracting the mean and dividing by the standard deviation. Since our proposed method uses 3D patches as input of the network, this operation could be done to each patch independently. However, since we use a sliding windows approach to denoise the images, we used a different approach to minimize block artifacts that could arise after mean restoration and standard deviation restoration.

First, we estimated a low-pass filtered image with a box-car kernel with the same size of the patch (local mean map). Second, we estimated local standard deviation map using the same patch size (local standard deviation map). Afterwards, these two images were used to normalize the input and output volumes by subtracting the local mean map and dividing by the local standard deviation map (see Fig. 1). We found that this approach introduces significantly less blocking artifacts than the standard approach.

2.3   Proposed Method

The proposed approach is based on a patch-wise single scale CNN (no max-pooling). The input and output of the proposed CNN are 3D patches of size $12 \times 12 \times 12$ voxels. Such patches are extracted from the pre-processed images in an over complete manner with an overlapping of 6 voxels in all three dimensions.

Differently from other approaches were different networks are trained to filter different levels of noise [10], our pre-processing fixes to approximately one the amount of noise present at each patch. Thanks to this, our network is able to blindly deal with arbitrary levels of noise and besides is naturally suited to deal with spatially variant noise levels which are quite common in modern MRIs.

Overcomplete Patch-Based CNN
The topology of the proposed network is the following. First, one input block of size $12 \times 12 \times 12$ composed of one 3D convolution and a RELU layer with 64 filters of $3 \times 3 \times 3$ voxels. Then, seven repeated blocks composed of a Batch-Normalization, a 3D convolution plus a RELU. Finally, a last block composed of a Batch Normalization and a 3D convolution to produces a $12 \times 12 \times 12$ output patch (see Fig. 1). To train the network we used ADAM optimizer, 100 epochs and a batch size of 128 patches. We used an early stop criterion using the validation data which represented the 10% of the training data. The whole network has a total of 779,009 trainable parameters.

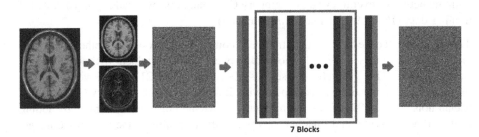

Fig. 1. 2D example of the proposed patch-based CNN model. Block design: Red (Batch Normalization), Blue (3D convolution) and Green (RELU). (Color figure online)

We used a residual learning approach (i.e., the network learns how to produce noise map) as in [10] instead of using residual connexions in the network (i.e., the residual network is trained to produce denoised image) as we found this option more effective (faster training and better results). Basically, instead of learning the noise-free patch, we learn the noise present in the patch. This is done by the network simply removing correlated information in the input layer. Differently from [10] where the network remove the original image from the input, our network starts with a pre-processed patch that is highly similar to the output patch. Therefore, the effort of the network to remove the anatomy is lower and the problem to solve easier.

We trained the network using around 300.000 patches randomly selected from the cases of each library (i.e. we trained a network using only patches from MNI dataset and one using only IXI dataset). We used the mean squared error as loss function. Once the network is trained, the test image (i.e., the Brainweb phantom) is filtered using an overcomplete 3D sliding window approach. This overcomplete approach further reduces the noise by averaging several overlapping estimations and contributes to reduce block artefacts.

Rotational Invariant Denoising
As shown in Manjón et al. [7], when a good quality pre-filtered image is available we can use this image within a rotationally invariant NLM filter to robustly perform a local similarity estimation defined as follow:

$$\widehat{A}(i) = \frac{\sum\limits_{j \in \Omega} w(i,j) y(i)}{\sum\limits_{j \in \Omega} w(i,j)} \qquad w(i,j) = e^{-\frac{1}{2}\left(\frac{(g(i)-g(j))^2 + 3(\mu_{N_i} - \mu_{N_j})^2}{2h_i^2}\right)} \qquad (2)$$

where μ_{Ni} and μ_{Nj} are the mean values of patches N_i and N_j around voxels i and j in the guide image g, h is related to the standard deviation of the noise present on image y and Ω represents position of the elements of the search volume. We refer the interested reader to the original paper [7] to see the full details of the rotational invariant NLM filter. Rician noise bias was removed as described in Manjón et al. [7].

It is worth noting that applying this rotational invariant NLM using the proposed CNN guide image not only outperforms the use of the CNN only but also helps to remove small remaining block artifacts.

3   Experiments and Results

In this section, a set of experiments are presented to show how the hyper parameters of the proposed network were selected and some comparisons with state-of-the-art methods. To evaluate the results, we used the Peak Signal to noise Ratio (PSNR) estimated between the denoised and the noise free Brainweb phantom.

3.1   Network Topology

We explored several options to design the proposed patch-based CNN, such as the patch-size, number of layers or the number of filters. For the number of filters, we tested 16, 32 and 64 filters, the results showed that the higher the number of filters the better the results. We chose 64 filters because 128 significantly increased the model size and training time but the improvement was modest. Regarding the number of layers, we found that increasing the number of layers to have a receptive field wider than the patch size was not improving significantly the results. We tested patch sizes of $6 \times 6 \times 6$, $12 \times 12 \times 12$ and $24 \times 24 \times 24$ voxels and we found that the best results were obtained for $12 \times 12 \times 12$ voxels (with 7 internal blocks covering a receptive field of $17 \times 17 \times 17$ voxels).

3.2   Impact of Training Data

We trained the designed network using the both described datasets (MNI and IXI) and compared the results on the Brainweb dataset used as testing dataset. We added Gaussian noise (range 1 to 9%) to these images to simulate noisy cases. We did not add Rician noise as the Rician bias correction is performed at postprocessing as described in [7]. We also evaluated the impact of the level of overlapping over the final results. Specifically, offsets of 6 and 3 voxels in all 3 dimensions were evaluated. The results are shown in Table 1.

As can be noted, the best results were obtained when using the IXI dataset. This was counter intuitive as we thought that the patterns of the synthetic MNI dataset and the Brainweb phantom being similar, the results would be better when using this dataset. We think that the patterns of the IXI dataset being richer and more complex allowed the network to better generalize. As expected, we found also that the higher the overlap the better the results (at the expense of a higher computational time, 17 vs 120 s).

Table 1. PSNR results on the Brainweb phantom for the proposed method for stationary Gaussian noise with two different training datasets (the MNI and IXI datasets).

Filter	Gaussian noise level					
	1%	3%	5%	7%	9%	Mean
Noisy	39.99	30.46	26.02	23.10	20.91	28.10
PB-CNN(MNI) offset = 6	45.46	39.82	37.26	35.38	33.91	38.36
PB-CNN(MNI) offset = 3	45.58	40.02	37.51	35.65	34.22	38.59
PB-CNN(IXI) offset = 6	45.49	40.46	37.89	36.14	34.78	38.95
PB-CNN(IXI) offset = 3	**45.82**	**40.70**	**38.18**	**36.44**	**35.10**	**39.24**

3.3   Methods Comparison

We compared our proposed method with other recent state of the art denoising methods. The compared methods are called PRI-NL-PCA [7], BM4D [12], MCDnCNNg (blind) and MCDnCNNs (several noise specific networks) [10] and the proposed method trained with IXI data. Both Gaussian and Rician noise with different levels were evaluated. Tables 2 and 3 summarize the results of the comparison.

As can be noticed, the combination of the proposed PB-CNN with the RI-NLM further improves the results for both stationary Gaussian and Rician noise. The proposed method outperformed the compared methods for all noise levels and noise types.

Table 2. PSNR results on the Brainweb phantom of the compared methods for stationary Gaussian noise.

Filter	Gaussian noise level					
	1%	3%	5%	7%	9%	Mean
Noisy	39.99	30.46	26.02	23.10	20.91	28.10
PRI-NL-PCA	45.38	39.33	36.63	34.90	33.58	37.96
BM4D	44.02	38.35	35.91	34.31	33.10	37.14
PB-CNN	45.82	40.70	38.18	36.44	35.10	39.24
PRI-PB-CNN	**47.13**	**41.43**	**38.77**	**37.03**	**35.65**	**40.00**

Table 3. PSNR results on the Brainweb phantom of the compared methods for stationary Rician noise. Results of MCDnCNNg and MCDnCNNg methods [10] were estimated from Fig. 6.

Filter	Rician noise level					
	1%	3%	5%	7%	9%	Mean
Noisy	40.00	30.49	26.09	23.20	21.04	28.16
PRI-NL-PCA	45.31	39.34	36.58	34.74	33.28	37.85
BM4D	44.09	38.35	35.84	34.17	32.88	36.99
MCDnCNNg	43.80	38.10	36.00	34.50	33.00	37.08
MCDnCNNs	45.20	39.80	37.20	35.20	33.50	38.18
PB-CNN	45.20	39.82	37.48	35.54	33.74	38.35
PRI-PB-CNN	**46.67**	**40.45**	**38.17**	**36.09**	**34.24**	**39.12**

3.4   Qualitative Evaluation on Real Images

Although the results on synthetic data are easy to interpret, they might by not realistic enough. To qualitatively evaluate the results of the proposed method we applied it to two real images and we evaluators visually the results. In Fig. 2 the results can be visually checked. As can be noticed, no anatomical information can be observed in the residuals. Finally, it is worth noting that a network trained on T1 images can be used to denoise T2 images effectively thanks to its patch-based nature.

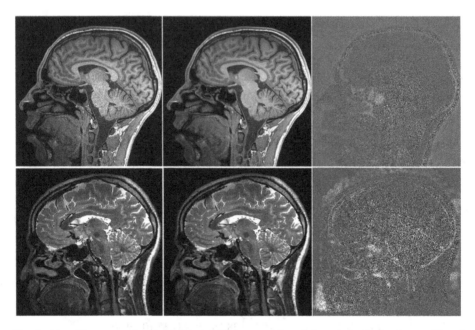

Fig. 2. Denoising example of real T1 and T2 images. From left to right: Noisy image, filtered image with the proposed filter and residual image (removed Rician noise).

4 Discussion

In this paper, we have presented a new method for MRI denoising that combines the benefits of new deep learning techniques with the strength of the traditional non-local image processing methods. The proposed method is based on an overcomplete patch-based CNN which produces a pre-filtered image which is used as a guide image within a rotational invariant non-local means framework.

The proposed method outperformed compared methods for all noise levels and noise types (Gaussian and Rician) and is an effective approach for automatically reduce the amount on noise in MR images in a blind manner thanks to its automatic adaptation to different levels of noise. Furthermore, although it was not designed to do so the proposed method is able to deal with spatially variant noise as can be noticed at Fig. 2 thanks to its adaptive patch-based nature.

Acknowledgements. This research was supported by the Spanish DPI2017-87743-R grant from the Ministerio de Economia, Industria y Competitividad of Spain. This study has been also carried out with financial support from the French State, managed by the French National Research Agency (ANR) in the frame of the Investments for the future Program IdEx Bordeaux (ANR-10-IDEX-03-02, HL-MRI Project) and Cluster of excellence CPU and TRAIL (HR-DTI ANR-10-LABX-57). The authors gratefully acknowledge the support of NVIDIA Corporation with their donation of the TITAN X GPU used in this research.

References

1. Mohan, J., Krishnaveni, V., Guo, Y.: A survey on the magnetic resonance image denoising methods. Biomed. Signal Process. Control **9**, 56–69 (2014)
2. Buades, A., Coll, B., Morel, J.M.: A non-local algorithm for image denoising. In: IEEE International Conference on Computer Vision and Pattern Recognition (CPVR), vol. 2, pp. 60–65 (2005)
3. Coupé, P., Yger, P., Prima, S., Hellier, P., Kervrann, C., Barillot, C.: An optimized blockwise nonlocal means denoising filter for 3-D magnetic resonance images. IEEE Trans. Med. Imaging **27**, 425–441 (2008)
4. Manjón, J.V., et al.: MRI denoising using non-local means. Med. Image Anal. **4**, 514–523 (2008)
5. He, L., Greenshields, I.R.: A nonlocal maximum likelihood estimation method for Rician noise reduction in MR images. IEEE Trans. Med. Imaging **28**, 165–172 (2009)
6. Guleryuz, O.G.: Weighted overcomplete denoising. In: Proceedings of the Asilomar Conference on Signals and Systems (2003)
7. Manjón, J.V., Coupé, P., Buades, A.: MRI noise estimation and denoising using non-local PCA. Med. Image Anal. **22**(1), 35–47 (2015)
8. Gondara, L.: Medical image denoising using convolutional denoising autoencoders. In: Proceedings of the ICDMW, pp. 241–246 (2016)
9. Benou, A., Veksler, R., Friedman, A., Riklin, R.T.: Ensemble of expert deep neural networks for spatio-temporal denoising of contrast-enhanced MRI sequences. Med. Image Anal. **42**, 145–159 (2017)
10. Jiang, D., Dou, W., Vosters, L., Xu, X., Sun, Y., Tan, T.: Denoising of 3D magnetic resonance images with multi-channel residual learning of convolutional neural network (2018). arXiv:1712.08726v2
11. Collins, D.L., et al.: Design and construction of a realistic digital brain phantom. IEEE Trans. Med. Imaging **17**, 463–468 (1998)
12. Maggioni, M., Katkovnik, V., Egiazarian, K., Foi, A.: Nonlocal transform-domain filter for volumetric data denoising and reconstruction. IEEE Trans. Image Process. **22**(1), 119–133 (2013)

MRI Denoising and Artefact Removal Using Self-Organizing Maps for Fast Global Block-Matching

Lee B. Reid[1]([envelope]) [ORCID], Ashley Gillman[1,2], Alex M. Pagnozzi[1] [ORCID],
José V. Manjón[3] [ORCID], and Jurgen Fripp[1] [ORCID]

[1] The Australian e-Health Research Centre, Commonwealth Scientific and Industrial
Research Organisation, Brisbane, QLD, Australia
lee.reid@csiro.au
[2] Faculty of Medicine, The University of Queensland, St Lucia, QLD, Australia
[3] Universitat Politècnia de València, ITACA, 46022 Valencia, Spain

Abstract. Image noise and motion degrade the quality of MR images.
Block-matching methods are a well-demonstrated means of improving
signal-to-noise ratios in such images. Ideally, block-matching methods
would search within the entire image for matching patches to a target, leveraging an image's full informational redundancy, but this car-
ries impractical computational costs. A well-known workaround, implemented in the traditional Non-Local Means (NLM) filter, is to search
for matching patches only within a local neighborhood. Here, we detail
a Global Approximate Block-matching (GAB) method that, via a self-
organizing map, rapidly searches an entire image for patches similar
to a target. Four sets of five T1 + five FLAIR images were acquired.
GAB and NLM both denoised the T1s; the results were compared to
subject-wise mean images with very low noise. GAB reliably produced
images that were more similar to these 'templates' than NLM. This was
repeated for the same images with motion-like artefacts artificially added.
GAB, again, outperformed NLM. For this task, GAB further improved
with multichannel inputs, even if the FLAIR image contained artefacts.
GAB's competitive performance appeared to be due to a better balance
between preserving image features and removing noise/artefacts. The
performance of GAB and NLM variants hinted that GAB's advantage
was not brute-force processing, but its ability to effectively search the
whole image.

Keywords: Block-matching · Self-organizing map · Image noise
MRI artefacts · Non-local means

1 Introduction

Images with motion artefacts and/or high levels of noise are an unfortunate real-
ity for many magnetic resonance projects and clinical facilities. Block-matching

© Crown Copyright is asserted by the Australian Government 2018
W. Bai et al. (Eds.): Patch-MI 2018, LNCS 11075, pp. 20–27, 2018.
https://doi.org/10.1007/978-3-030-00500-9_3

(BM) techniques are typically designed to remove such noise. These methods typically accept a single input image, match similar cubes of voxels (patches) to one another, and compute a weighted average according to the patch similarity. This approach is known as 'non-local means' [2]. BM leverages the small patterns that exist throughout an image, such as the repeated folding of brain tissue. BM techniques are unable to take full advantage of this redundancy, however, because exhaustively comparing patches to one another is extremely computationally expensive. To circumvent this, many patch-based techniques such as the traditional non-local means method [3,4], herein referred to as 'NLM', search only a selected local area for patches similar to a target, assuming that most of the pattern redundancy is local.

An alternative, or complementary, way to reduce this computational cost is through dimensionality reduction. The self-organizing map (SOM) is a flexible non-linear dimensionality reduction technique [5]. Briefly, SOMs are implemented as collection of nodes which each have local connectivity, a fixed position in low dimensional space (e.g. forming a 2D grid), and a trainable position in the high-dimensional space. SOMs train quickly through competitive learning, in a manner that results in a smooth projection between the two spaces. Intuitively, a trained 1D SOM can be thought of as optimally 'snaking' through high-dimensional space, much as principal components analysis (PCA) draws a straight line through such a space.

We have developed a 'Global Approximate Block-matching' algorithm (GAB) which performs a whole-image search for patches matching each target. To reduce this operation's computational burden, GAB collapses each patch into a singular value (SV) through a dimensionality reduction method such as the SOM, which allows binary search lookups. Here, we describe GAB and demonstrate its use for removal of noise and motion artefacts in T1 images, utilizing both single- (T1) and multi-channel (T1 + FLAIR) input data. Performances of four variants of GAB are compared to that of NLM.

2   Methods

2.1   Overview

We tested the ability of GAB and NLM to perform two related tasks: (1) reduction of noise, and (2) removal of motion artefacts. Images used were acquired from a modern scanner, with simulated motion artefacts added for the second task. Performance was measured by the quantitative similarity between the processed T1 image and a low-noise template that was an average of five scans of the same subject.

2.2   Global Approximate Block Matching and Comparator Methods

GAB can run in single- or multi-channel mode, and is summarized in Fig. 1. To conserve memory, input image(s) are linearly scaled and voxel intensities stored

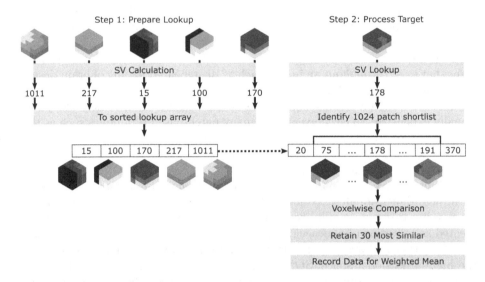

Fig. 1. In Step 1 (top left), the image was split into overlapping $3 \times 3 \times 3$ voxel patches, or $3 \times 3 \times 3 \times 2$ voxel patches in the case of dual-channel processing. For each patch, a singular value (SV) was calculated using one of four methods. Patches were then sorted by these SVs. In Step 2, for each target patch, the 1024 atlas patches with the most similar SVs were selected (the 'shortlist'). The voxelwise sum of square differences (SSD) was calculated for these patches versus the target, and the 30 patches with the lowest SSDs selected to contribute toward final image reconstruction. See the text for details on final image reconstruction.

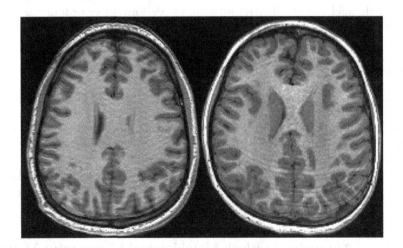

Fig. 2. T1 MPRAGE images with simulated (left) and real motion artefacts (right), acquired with the same sequence and scanner.

as 8-bit integers. The image within the brain mask is split into overlapping $3 \times 3 \times 3$ voxel patches ($3 \times 3 \times 3 \times$ n-channels for multi-channel mode). A SV is calculated for each patch (see below), by which patches are then sorted. During denoising, the location of a target patch can be found through a simple SV-indexed binary search. A 1024 patch shortlist is then identified as those items from 512 positions before to 511 indices after this index. The voxelwise sum of square differences (SSD) is calculated between the target patch and shortlist, excluding the original patch itself, identifying the 30 most similar patches to the target. These patches are each multiplied by their weight ($1/(SSD + 10^{-6})$), filtered by a Gaussian of $\sigma = 1$ voxel, and (all 27 voxels per weighted patch) are added to a 'sum' image. These weights, also multiplied by this Gaussian are added to a 'weights' image. Upon completion of all block matching, the sum image is divided by the weights image to generate a final reconstruction. This non-intuitive unweighting is required because each voxel in the 'sum' image is contributed to by up to 27 block-matching operations, each operation in turn averaging 30 weighted patches from the shortlist.

SVs were calculated solely from voxel intensities. Here, four SV methods were compared: PCA (ϵ_0), mean intensity, random (SV randomly generated), and SOM. PCA and SOM training sets were up to 10^7 patches randomly selected from the input image. Each SOM was arranged as a 1D array of 4096 equally-spaced nodes. Training took 10–40 s for a single-channel input. SV calculation using the SOM was performed by locating a patch's continuous position in this array (i.e. between the best matched node and its most similar neighbor) based on voxelwise SSD.

For a comparator method, we utilized NLM with a Rician noise model [3,4], as implemented in DIPY. This is single-channel and utilizes $3 \times 3 \times 3$ voxel patches. Two search radii were tested: 5 voxels (728 patches; the default setting; NLM-5) and 6 voxels (1330 patches; NLM-6). Other settings were left as default.

2.3 Dataset

Four adults (28–32y) were scanned on a 3T Siemens Prisma. MPRAGE and FLAIR images (both $1\,mm^3$ resolution) were acquired in an alternating fashion. Five of each were acquired per subject. Noise and intensity biases can vary within an image, due in part to voxels' differing locations within the B0 field and proximity to the head coil. We wished to reduce the likelihood of images displaying local intensity biases, or higher noise levels, at consistent anatomical locations, so as to generate more representative 'ground truth' (template) images (see below). As such, subjects reoriented their head before each T1 acquisition. The field of view was coarsely adjusted each time only to ensure that the full head was contained within the image. Subjects remained still during acquisition and gave written informed consent. Ethical approval was granted through the Herston Imaging Research Facility. All acquired images were N4 bias corrected [6] and linearly intensity scaled such that 95% of non-zero voxels were within the range of 1–100, prior to all processing and analysis.

Low Noise Template. For each subject, a low noise template T1 was generated as follows: (1) the aforementioned bias-corrected and intensity normalized images were upsampled to $0.5\,mm^3$ with trilinear interpolation; (2) an initial mean image was calculated, and brainmask generated by affine transforming the FSL MNI 152 T1 brainmask into this space using ANTS [1]; (3) each interpolated image was rigid-registered to the mean (from its original orientation) using ANTS; (4) another mean was then calculated. Steps 3 and 4 were repeated four times, the final mean constituting the 'template' for that subject. These templates exhibited a very low level of noise (Fig. 3). Regarding Step 1, upsampling was performed to compensate for the interpolation effects later during resampling to target image space. A final brainmask was generated for each by affine transforming the FSL MNI 152 T1 brainmask into this space using ANTS.

Motion Corruption. In this work, motion corruption was simulated as head rotation around a central point. To do so, we manipulated images in Fourier space, to represent partial filling of k-space at two head orientations. Although many factors contribute to image reconstruction, this method provided sufficiently-realistic artefacts for the purpose of testing artefact removal. An example of artificial motion corruption is provided in Fig. 2.

We generated a motion-corrupted copy of each acquired bias-corrected image (I.E. five T1 and five FLAIR images per subject). This center of rotation was defined in voxel space as the position between the two thalami on the mid (i.e. third) image acquired for each subject. As subjects were reoriented between scans, this meant that the anatomical center of rotation differed in each image whilst still being at an anatomically-plausible location. Motion corrupted images were constructed by combining Fourier space data from unaltered images with that from images that had been rotated in image space. T1 and FLAIR images were rotated by ($5°$, $1°$, and $1°$) and ($1°$, $2°$, and $2°$), respectively, to give non-correlated motion. After an FFT, these rotated images were multiplied by two to ensure a moderate artefact effect. Real and imaginary T1 images were constructed by combining coronal-planes 0–80 of the rotated data with 81–175 of the original image. Real and imaginary FLAIR images, which were acquired a different plane to our T1 images, were constructed from sagittal planes 0–70 of the rotated data and 71–191 of the original image. An FFT then reconstructed these data back into image space.

2.4 Performance Metric

Each BM method performed two sets of tasks: (1) reduction of noise in T1 images and (2) removal of the aforementioned motion artefacts from T1 images. For *noise reduction,* NLM accepted a single input image (T1). GAB was run with both a single-channel input (T1) and with multi-channel (T1+FLAIR) input. For *motion artefact* removal, NLM again accepted a single input image (corrupted T1), whilst GAB was run with single-channel (corrupted T1), multi-channel (corrupted T1 + FLAIR) and double-corrupted multichannel (corrupted T1 +

corrupted FLAIR) inputs. In all multi-channel conditions, analyses were run for the 25 possible combinations of T1 + FLAIR image pairs for each subject. For these conditions, FLAIR images were rigid-registered to the T1 using ANTS [1].

To calculate error, the high-resolution template for the appropriate subject was rigid registered to the target ('noise' or 'artefact' containing) T1 using ANTS [1] and resampled to 1 mm, providing voxelwise correspondence between images. BM-processed T1s were linearly scaled to match the histogram of this template image. The mean squared error (MSE) of image intensities was calculated between these processed images and their template within the template's brain-mask. Identical templates, registrations, and target images were used for each method. All registrations were visually checked.

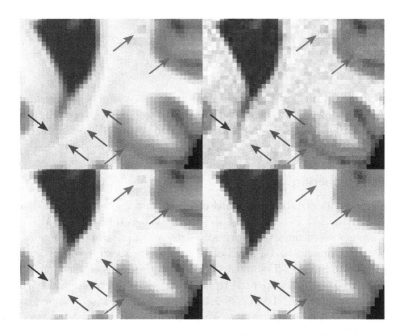

Fig. 3. Representative images of a template (top left); target bias-corrected T1 (top right); denoised result from single-channel GAB-SOM (bottom left); and denoised result from NLM performed with default settings (bottom right). Images are cropped to the brain mask. Note how GAB preserves image features such as sulci, the ventricular shape (green arrow) and intensities of structures including the optic radiation (blue arrows). (Color figure online)

3   Results

Tests were run on a single Tesla P100 GPU, 10 cores of a Xeon E5-2690 v4 compute node, and 64 GB of RAM. GAB was run on Mono 4.6.2 and OpenCL 1.2. NLM ran through a Python 2.7.13 wrapper for compiled code. The mean

Table 1. Mean MSE ± SD across all subjects, for each of the tested methods and conditions. The left two columns reflect denoising; the right three reflect artefact removal. The best denoising and artefact removal scores are highlighted. Abbreviations: MC, Motion Corrupted; NLM-5, traditional Non-Local Means (search radius = 5); NLM-6, traditional Non-Local Means (search radius = 6); PCA, Principal Components Analysis; GAB, Global Approximate Block Matching; SOM, Self-Organizing Map.

Method	Noise reduction		Motion artefact removal		
	T1	T1+FLAIR	MC T1	MC T1 + FLAIR	MC T1 + MC FLAIR
GAB-SOM	**4.3 ± 1.7**	6.0 ± 1.2	14.2 ± 1.1	**12.3 ± 1.0**	12.9 ± 1.0
GAB-Mean	5.8 ± 1.5	11.0 ± 1.0	14.4 ± 1.2	15.8 ± 1.3	16.4 ± 1.3
GAB-PCA	6.4 ± 1.4	13.5 ± 1.3	15.2 ± 1.4	18.1 ± 1.7	18.9 ± 1.7
NLM-5	7.3 ± 1.7	N/A	16.5 ± 1.4	N/A	N/A
NLM-6	7.7 ± 1.6	N/A	16.4 ± 1.4	N/A	N/A
GAB-Random	16.4 ± 6.7	28.8 ± 6.8	21.1 ± 3.9	30.8 ± 8.1	30.0 ± 7.3
No Correction	12.1 ± 2.0	12.1 ± 2.0	26.8 ± 1.8	26.8 ± 1.8	26.8 ± 1.8

run time (of all variants) of GAB was 247 s for single-channel processing; GAB-SOM was ∼30 s slower than other variants. Multi-channel processing increased run times by ∼100% for GAB-SOM and ∼30% for other SV methods. NLM ran in 40 s and 70 s on average for radii of 5 and 6 voxels, respectively.

3.1 Noise Reduction

Twenty single-channel, and 100 multi-channel, tests were conducted and are summarized in the left two columns of Table 1. When interpreting MSE values, note that images were intensity normalized to an approximate range of 0–100. Non-denoised T1 images had a MSE of 12.14 ± 2.00 (Mean ± SD), compared to their respective templates. The most effective method was single-channel GAB-SOM (4.24 ± 1.65), which appeared to better balance noise removal with image feature preservation than NLM (7.29 ± 1.66; Fig. 3). NLM performance was not bolstered by a greater search radius. Multi-channel GAB provided poorer performance than single-channel GAB.

3.2 Artefact Removal

One motion-corrupted T1 image was unable to be registered with its template, and was discarded, resulting in 19 T1s contributing to 19 single-channel, and 95 multi-channel, tests. Results are summarized in the right three columns of Table 1. Corrupted T1 images showed a MSE of 26.83 ± 1.75 (Mean ± SD). Single channel GAB-SOM (14.20 ± 1.07), GAB-Mean, and GAB-PCA, outperformed NLM (16.39 ± 1.38). Qualitatively, NLM often appeared to better reduce this artefact, but again this came at the expense of modification or deletion of features apparent in the template image. Including FLAIR data substantially improved GAB-SOM effectiveness (12.34 ± 1.00), even if the FLAIR image contained artefacts (12.86 ± 0.98).

3.3 Discussion

We proposed a BM method that initially performs a rapid global search for a shortlist of approximately similar patches that are to be compared voxelwise to a target. Ultimately, GAB, performed more accurately and reliably than NLM in removing image artefacts and noise, whilst preserving image features (Table 1; Fig. 3). NLM executed faster than GAB, but GAB's run time of $\sim$3–8 min is still well within acceptable bounds for image preprocessing. Although we relied on artificial motion-like artefacts, these artefacts were a fair approximation of the genuine artefacts we see in our facility (Fig. 2). It is unlikely that any shortcomings in our simulation biased results as BM methods were not optimized for motion artefacts, nor particular sequences or scanners.

In single-channel mode, GAB's advantage appeared to be primarily due to its better leveraging of image redundancies, rather than brute force computation. This is indicated by its poor performance when patch shortlists were random, and the lesser performance of NLM even when performing 30% more voxelwise comparisons than GAB (NLM-6). GAB performed more poorly when denoising a good-quality T1 in multichannel mode than when that T1 was the only input. Results for GAB-Random implied that this may be due to inappropriate scaling of patch weighting factors (1/SSD), given such a high-dimensional space, and/or the FLAIR image being interpolated during reslicing to T1 space. When processing images with artefacts, however, multichannel information improved the performance of GAB-SOM, even with mild artefacts in the FLAIR image. Here, the SOM's non-linearity presumably enabled a meaningful 54-to-1 dimensionality reduction, given the substantially poorer results of GAB-PCA.

In conclusion, we proposed a global approximate BM method that uses a SOM for dimensionality reduction. In real images this outperformed traditional NLM when removing both image noise and simulated motion artefacts.

References

1. Avants, B.B., Epstein, C.L., Grossman, M., Gee, J.C.: Symmetric diffeomorphic image registration with cross-correlation: evaluating automated labeling of elderly and neurodegenerative brain. Med. Image Anal. **12**(1), 26–41 (2008)
2. Buades, A., Coll, B., Morel, J.M.: A non-local algorithm for image denoising. In: 2005 IEEE Computer Society Conference on Computer Vision and Pattern Recognition, vol. 2, pp. 60–65. IEEE (2005)
3. Coupé, P., Manjón, J., Robles, M., Collins, D.: Adaptive multiresolution non-local means filter for three-dimensional magnetic resonance image denoising. IET Image Process. **6**(5), 558 (2012)
4. Coupé, P., Yger, P., Prima, S., Hellier, P., Kervrann, C., Barillot, C.: An optimized blockwise nonlocal means denoising filter for 3-D magnetic resonance images. IEEE Trans. Med. Imaging **27**(4), 425–441 (2008)
5. Kohonen, T.: Self-organized formation of topologically correct feature maps. Biol. Cybern. **43**(1), 59–69 (1982)
6. Tustison, N.J., et al.: N4ITK: improved N3 bias correction. IEEE Trans. Med. Imaging **29**(6), 1310–20 (2010)

A Monte Carlo Framework for Denoising and Missing Wedge Reconstruction in Cryo-electron Tomography

E. Moebel$^{(\boxtimes)}$ and C. Kervrann

Inria Rennes - Bretagne Atlantique, Campus universitaire de Beaulieu,
35042 Rennes Cedex, France
emmanuel.moebel@inria.fr

Abstract. We propose a statistical method to address an important issue in cryo electron tomography image analysis: reduction of a high amount of noise and artifacts due to the presence of a missing wedge (MW) in the spectral domain. The method takes as an input a 3D tomogram derived from limited-angle tomography, and gives as an output a 3D denoised and artifact compensated tomogram. The artifact compensation is achieved by filling up the MW with meaningful information. The method can be used to enhance visualization or as a pre-processing step for image analysis, including segmentation and classification. Results are presented for both synthetic and experimental data.

Keywords: Cryo electron tomography · Patch-based denoising
Missing wedge restoration · Stochastic models · Monte Carlo simulation

1 Introduction

Cryo electron tomography (cryo-ET) is intended to explore the structure of an entire cell and constitutes a rapidly growing field in biology. The particularity of cryo-ET is that it is able to produce near to atomic resolution three-dimensional views of vitrified samples, which allows observing the structure of molecular complexes (e.g. ribosomes) in their physiological environment. This precious insight in the mechanism of a cell comes with a cost: i/ due to the low dose of electrons used to preserve specimen integrity during image acquisition, the amount of noise is very high; ii/ due to technical limitations of the microscope, complete tilting of the sample (180°) is impossible, resulting into a blind spot. In other words, projections are not available for a determined angle range, hence the term "limited angle tomography". This blind spot is observable in the Fourier domain, where the missing projections appear as a missing wedge (MW). This separates the Fourier spectrum into: the sampled region (SR) and the unsampled regions (MW). The sharp transition between these two regions is responsible for a Gibbs-like phenomenon: ray- and side-artifacts emanate from high contrast objects (see Fig. 1), which can hide important structural features in the image.

© Springer Nature Switzerland AG 2018
W. Bai et al. (Eds.): Patch-MI 2018, LNCS 11075, pp. 28–35, 2018.
https://doi.org/10.1007/978-3-030-00500-9_4

Another type of artifact arises from the incomplete angular sampling: objects appear elongated in the blind spot's direction (see Fig. 1). This elongation erases boundaries and makes it difficult to differentiate neighboring features.

Filling up the MW with relevant data can reduce or completely suppress these artifacts. Experimentally this can partially be done using dual-axis tomography [4], where the sample is tilted with respect to the second axis. Consequently the blind spot is smaller and the MW becomes a missing pyramid, which results into a smaller missing spectrum. In practice dual-axis tomography is technically more difficult to achieve and requires intensive post-processing in order to correct tilt and movement bias in the microscope. Another strategy consists in exploiting the symmetry of the observed structure to fill up the MW [3], but this can only be applicable to specific structures (e.g. virus). Another technique consists in combining several images, each containing a different instance of the same object, but with distinct blind spots. This technique is routinely used in cryo-ET and is known as sub-tomogram averaging [3], but it relies on the acquisition of several views of the same object type. Accordingly, edicated tomographic reconstruction algorithms have also been proposed, to compensate MW artifacts by using a regularization term [7,10] and exploiting prior information. A simpler way of handling MW artifacts is described in [6], where a spectral filter is used to smooth out the transition between the SR and the MW. This filter is thus able to reduce ray- and side-artifacts, but the object elongation remains.

In this paper, we propose a stochastic method inspired from [2] for restoring 2D images and adapted to 3D in [9], and re-interpret the method to recover the MW in cryo-ET from a Monte Carlo (MC) sampling perspective. The method [9] has been shown to successfully recover missing regions in the Fourier domain, achieving excellent results for several missing region shapes, including the MW shape. The method [9] works by alternatively adding noise into the missing region and applying a patch-based denoising algorithm (BM4D). However, the method has no clear theoretical framework and appears therefore empirical. The authors interpret their method as a compressed sensing algorithm, which relies on two conditions: sparsity of the signal in some transform, and the incoherence between this transform and the sampling matrix. Actually, BM4D does rely on a transform where the signal is sparse. Nevertheless, it is not clearly established that this transform is incoherent with the sampling matrix, defined by the support of the SR. Therefore, there is no theoretical proof of convergence, even though the authors show numerical convergence. Also, the data in [9] is exclusively synthetic and corrupted with white Gaussian noise, for which BM4D has been well designed. It remains unclear how the method performs with experimental data and non Gaussian noise.

Consequently, we reformulate the method [9] as a Metropolis-Hastings procedure in the MCMC framework (Sect. 2), and demonstrate that it performs as well as the original method but converges faster. Moreover, any patch-based denoiser can be applied [5,8,9] and the concept is more general than [9]. Finally, we provide evidence that our method enhances signal in experimental cryo electron tomography images (Sect. 3).

2 Statistical and Computational Approach

Formally, we denote Y the n-dimensional noisy image, and $X \in \mathbb{R}^n$ the unknown image where $n = |\Omega|$ is the number of pixels of the volume Ω. We consider the following observation model:

$$Y = \mathcal{M}(X + \eta) \tag{1}$$

where $\eta \sim \mathcal{N}(0, I_{n \times n}\sigma_e^2)$ is a white Gaussian noise, $I_{n \times n}$ is the n-dimensional identity matrix, and $\mathcal{M}(.)$ is an operator setting to zero the Fourier coefficients belonging to the MW support.

To recover the unknown image, we propose a dedicated Monte-Carlo sampling procedure that generates at each iteration k a sample $\hat{X}_k \in \mathbb{R}^n$ (see Fig. 2). This procedure is based on the Metropolis-Hastings algorithm, determined by two steps: i/ a proposal step, where a n-dimensional candidate image is generated from a proposal distribution; ii/ an evaluation step, where the candidate is either accepted or rejected according to the Gibbs energy $E(\hat{X}_k)$, defined as the l_2 norm between the candidate $\hat{X}_k$ and the observed image Y:

$$E(\hat{X}_k) = \| \mathcal{M}(Y) - \mathcal{M}(\hat{X}_k) \|^2 . \tag{2}$$

In addition, we compute the norm on the SR support only, given that the MW of Y contains no information.

Formally, the procedure is defined as follows:

1. **PROPOSAL STEP:**
   - **Perturbation:** we perturb the current $\hat{X}_k$ with a n-dimensional white Gaussian noise with variance σ_p^2: $\hat{X}_k^\epsilon = \hat{X}_k + \epsilon$, with $\epsilon \sim \mathcal{N}(0, I_{n \times n}\sigma_p^2)$.
   - **Projection:** we project $\hat{X}_k^\epsilon$ on the subspace of images having the same observed frequencies as Y: $\Pi(\hat{X}_k^\epsilon) = \mathrm{FT}^{-1}(I_S \times \mathrm{FT}(Y)) + (1 - I_S) \times \mathrm{FT}(\hat{X}_k^\epsilon))$ where FT denotes the Fourier transform, and I_S is a binary mask having values of 1 for Fourier coefficients belonging to the SR and values of 0 otherwise.
   - **Denoising:** $DN(\Pi(\hat{X}_k^\epsilon)) = \tilde{X}_k$.

2. **EVALUATION STEP:**
   Define $\hat{X}_{k+1}$ as:

$$\hat{X}_k = \begin{cases} \tilde{X}_k & \text{if } \alpha \leq \exp \dfrac{-\Delta E(\tilde{X}_k, \hat{X}_{k-1})}{\beta}, \\ \hat{X}_{k-1} & \text{otherwise,} \end{cases} \tag{3}$$

where α is a random variable: $\alpha \sim U[0,1]$ (uniform distribution), $\beta > 0$ is a scaling parameter and $\Delta E(\tilde{X}_k, \hat{X}_{k-1}) = E(\tilde{X}_k) - E(\hat{X}_{k-1})$.

Actually, the originality of our approach lies in the way the candidates are proposed. The objective is to explore a subset $\mathcal{S}$ of plausible images, $\mathcal{S}$ being shaped by our prior knowledge. The perturbation allows to randomly explore the image space around $\hat{X}_k$, applying the prior guaranties that the exploration is limited to $\mathcal{S}$. The prior is twofold: i/ the images should have the same SR as Y, hence the projection operation; ii/ the images should be piece-wise smooth and self-similar, hence the patch-based denoising.

In the Bayesian framework, we focus on the conditional expectation estimator, computed as the average of N generated samples $\hat{X}_k$:

$$\hat{X} = \lim_{N \to \infty} \frac{1}{N - N_b} \sum_{k=N_b}^{N} \hat{X}_k \simeq \frac{1}{Z} \sum_{\lambda=1}^{M} e^{-E(X_\lambda)} X_\lambda \qquad (4)$$

where Z is a normalization constant and M is the cardinal of the space $\mathcal{S}$ of admissible images. It is recommended to introduce a burn-in phase to get a more satisfying estimator. Hence, the first N_b samples are discarded in the average $\hat{X}$.

In the end, the method is governed by three parameters: the number of iterations N, the noise variance σ_n^2 and the scaling parameter β. At each iteration k, the patch-based denoising algorithm removes the perturbation noise ϵ. The parameter β affects the acceptance rate of the evaluation step. The higher the value of β, the higher the acceptance rate. For a high enough β value, all proposed samples are accepted and we fall back on the original method [9]. This method cannot retrieve unobserved data, but it merely makes the best statistical guess of what the missing data could be, based on what has been observed.

This iterative procedure is successful provided that the denoising algorithm is able to remove the perturbation noise. In practice, the perturbation noise is Gaussian, as most of state-of-the-art denoising algorithm assume additive white Gaussian noise. This also means that any performant denoising algorithms including BM4D can be used in this framework [1,5,8]. Depending on the image contents and modality, some denoising methods could be more adapted than others, given their particular properties and assumptions.

3   Experimental Results

In this section, we present the results when the denoising is performed by using BM4D and $\sigma_e = \sigma_n$ in order to compare to [9]. We considered $N = 1000$ iterations and a burn-in phase of $K_b = 100$ iterations. Similar results have been obtained with the patch-based denoiser NL-Bayes [8].

Data Description. Three data sets (A, B and C) have been used to evaluate the performance of the method. Dataset A has been simulated, and consists of a density map of the 20S proteasome, first corrupted by adding varying amount of noise and then by applying artificially the MW (by giving zero-values to Fourier coefficients using a wedge shaped mask). Dataset B is an experimental sub-tomogram containing a gold particle. Dataset C is an experimental sub-tomogram containing 80S ribosomes attached to a membrane.

Evaluation Procedure. The evaluation differs depending on the dataset. For dataset A we have at our disposal a ground truth. We can thus use similarity measures like the PSNR (peak signal to noise ratio) for evaluation. In dataset B, we see that the gold particle is elongated (ellipse) due to the MW artefacts. Improving the sphericity of the object is thus a good evaluation criterion. For dataset C, we measure the similarity between the central ribosome and a reference (obtained via sub-tomogram averaging). The evaluation criterion is the Fourier shell correlation (FSC), commonly used in cryo-ET [11]. In order to measure the quality of the recovered MW only, we also compute the FSC over the MW support ("constrained" FSC or cFSC).

Results and Discussion. From the results on dataset A (Fig. 3(a)) it can be seen how well the method works in the absence of noise ($\sigma_n = 0$): a quasi perfect image recovery has been achieved, despite the complexity of the object. Increasing the amount of noise deteriorates the performance, but as can be observed for $\sigma_n = 0.2$ the result is still satisfying. For high amounts of noise ($\sigma_n = 0.4$), the object contrast is still greatly enhanced but the MW artifacts could not be completely removed. Let us examine the Fourier domain (Fig. 3(b)): in the absence of noise, the MW has been filled up completely, whereas for an increasing amount of noise the MW reconstruction is increasingly restrained to the low frequencies. This is because high frequency components of a signal are more affected by noise, which makes them more difficult to recover. In Fig. 3(c), the evolution of the PSNR over time shows that the method converges to a stable solution. In Fig. 3(d) we compare our method to the original one [9]. Both methods produce visually identical results in the spatial domain, as well as in the spectral domain, as can be confirmed by the final achieved PSNR values. However, the difference lies in convergence speed: our method takes about half as long as the original method [9]. Even though the synthetic dataset A is a simplified case of data corruption in cryo-EM, it gives a good intuition of the method performance.

The result on dataset B shows that noise is reduced and a significant part of the MW could be recovered (see Fig. 1). Even though the recovery is not complete, it is enough to reduce the MW artifacts while preserving and enhancing image details. The ray and side artifacts induced by the high contrast of the gold particle are reduced and its sphericity has been improved, bringing the image closer to the expected object shape. The result on this dataset shows that the method is able to handle experimental noise in cryo-ET.

The dataset C contains molecules (ribosomes) that have more interest for biologists (see Fig. 4). This case is more challenging, because the objects have a more complex shape and less contrast, i.e. the SNR is lower. Nonetheless, the method could enhance the contrast and according to the FSC criteria, the signal has indeed been improved. Although visually it is more difficult to conclude that the MW artifacts have been affected, the Fourier spectrum shows that Fourier coefficients could be recovered. With no surprise, the amount of recovered high frequencies is less than for dataset B, because of the lower SNR. It is now necessary to provide a proof that the recovered coefficients carry a coherent signal, therefore the cFSC has been measured. The black curve in Fig. 4 depicts the cFSC between the unprocessed image and the reference: given that the MW contains no information, the curve represents noise correlation. Consequently,

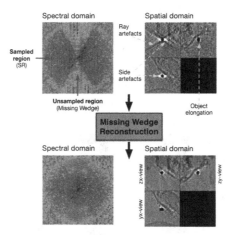

Fig. 1. Experimental sub-tomogram ($61 \times 61 \times 61$ voxels) containing a gold particle (dataset B). The top row shows the input in the spectral and spatial domains, the bottom row shows the output.

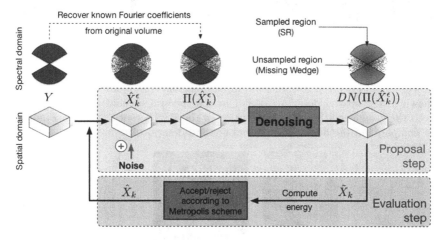

Fig. 2. The method flowchart. The 1st icon row represents the data in the spectral domain, the 2nd in the spatial domain.

everything above the black curve is signal, which is indeed the case for the processed data (red curve in Fig. 4). To illustrate how the method can improve visualization, a simple thresholding has been performed on the data (3D views in Fig. 4). While it is difficult to distinguish objects in the unprocessed data, the shape of ribosomes become clearly visible and it can be observed how they are fixated to the membrane.

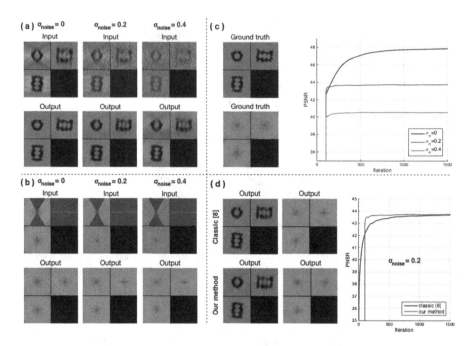

Fig. 3. Simulated data of the 20 S proteasome, for varying amounts of noise (dataset A). All images depict ortho-slices of 3D volumes. The volume size is 64 × 64 × 64 voxels. For (a) and (b), top row: method inputs, bottom row: method outputs. Results are shown in the spatial domain (a) and in the spectral domain (b). In (c) can be observed the ground truth and the evolution of the PSNR over iterations. Finally, in (d) we compare our method to the orginal method described in [9]

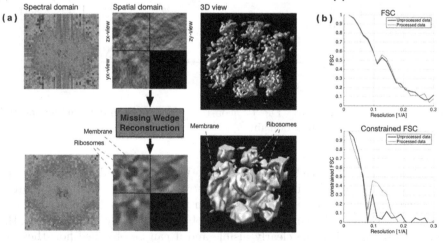

Fig. 4. Experimental sub-tomogram (46 × 46 × 46 voxels) containing ribosomes attached to a membrane (dataset C). (a) Top row: input image in spectral domain, spatial domain and 3D view of the thresholded data. Bottom row: the same representations for the output. (b) FSC and cFSC measures of the method input (in black) and output (in red). All measures are wrt the same reference. (Color figure online)

4   Conclusion

We have proposed a Monte-Carlo simulation method to denoise and compensate MW artifacts in cryo-ET images. Any patch-based denoiser can be used in this framework and the procedure converges faster than [9]. Our experiments on both synthetic and experimental data show that even for high amounts of noise, the method is able to enhance the signal. However, the method needs a reasonable constrast of the object of interest to perform well, which is not always the case in cryo-ET. Nevertheless, with improving electron microscopy techniques like direct electron detection sensors and phase contrast methods, the method will be able to produce even more impressive results. The effectiveness of the method being demonstrated for the challenging case of cryo-ET, the method can be applied to other imaging modalities, especially on images with high SNR values.

References

1. Buades, A., Coll, B., Morel, J.M.: A non-local algorithm for image denoising. Comput. Vis. Pattern Recognit. **2**, 60–65 (2005)
2. Egiazarian, K., Foi, A., Katkovnic, V.: Compressed sensing image reconstruction via recursive spatially adaptive filtering. Int. Conf. Image Process. **1**, 549–552 (2007)
3. Foerster, F., Hegerl, R.: Structure determination In Situ by averaging of tomograms. Cell. Electron Microsc. **79**, 741–767 (2007)
4. Guesdon, A., Blestel, S., Kervrann, C., Chrétien, D.: Single versus dual-axis cryo-electron tomography of microtubules assembled in vitro: limits and perspectives. J. Struct. Biol. **181**(2), 169–78 (2013)
5. Kervrann, C.: PEWA: patch-based exponentially weighted aggregation for image denoising. Adv. Neural Inf. Process. Syst. **27**, 1–9 (2014)
6. Kováčik, L., Kereïche, S., Höög, J.L., Jda, P., Matula, P., Raška, I.: A simple Fourier filter for suppression of the missing wedge ray artefacts in single-axis electron tomographic reconstructions. J. Struct. Biol. **186**(1), 141–52 (2014)
7. Leary, R., Saghi, Z., Midgley, P.A., Holland, D.J.: Compressed sensing electron tomography. Ultramicroscopy **131**, 70–91 (2013)
8. Lebrun, M., Buades, A., Morel, J.: A nonlocal Bayesian image denoising algorithm. SIAM J. Imaging Sci. **6**(3), 1665–1688 (2013)
9. Maggioni, M., Katkovnic, V., Egiazarian, K., Foi, A.: Nonlocal transform-domain filter for volumetric data denoising and reconstruction. IEEE Trans. Image Process. **22**(1), 119–133 (2013)
10. Paavolainen, L., et al.: Compensation of missing wedge effects with sequential statistical reconstruction in electron tomography. PLoS ONE **9**(10), 1–23 (2014)
11. Van Heel, M., Schatz, M.: Fourier shell correlation threshold criteria. J. Struct. Biol. **151**, 250–262 (2005)

Image Registration and Matching

Robust Supervoxel Matching Combining Mid-Level Spectral and Context-Rich Features

Florian Tilquin[1], Pierre-Henri Conze[2,3](✉), Patrick Pessaux[4],
Mathieu Lamard[3,5], Gwenolé Quellec[3], Vincent Noblet[1], and Fabrice Heitz[1]

[1] ICube UMR 7357, Université de Strasbourg, CNRS, FMTS, Strasbourg, France
`tilquin@unistra.fr`
[2] IMT Atlantique, Brest, France
`pierre-henri.conze@imt-atlantique.fr`
[3] Inserm, LaTIM UMR 1101, Brest, France
[4] Institut Hospitalo-Universitaire de Strasbourg, Strasbourg, France
[5] Université de Bretagne Occidentale, Brest, France

Abstract. This paper presents an innovative way to reach accurate semi-dense registration between images based on robust matching of structural entities. The proposed approach relies on a decomposition of images into visual primitives called supervoxels generated by aggregating adjacent voxels sharing similar characteristics. Two new categories of features are estimated at the supervoxel extent: mid-level spectral features relying on a spectral method applied on supervoxel graphs to capture the non-linear modes of intensity displacements, and mid-level context-rich features describing the broadened spatial context on the resulting spectral representations. Accurate supervoxel pairings are established by nearest neighbor search on these newly designed features. The effectiveness of the approach is demonstrated against state-of-the-art methods for semi-dense longitudinal registration of abdominal CT images, relying on liver label propagation and consistency assessment.

Keywords: Semi-dense image registration · Supervoxel matching
Mid-level representation · Laplacian graph · Spectral decomposition
Context-rich features

1 Introduction

Image registration is a crucial task in medical image analysis for organ motion compensation, longitudinal tumor follow-up, pre- and post-operative image matching or cohort analysis [1]. When coupled with a segmentation task through label transmission, it can usefully reduce the number of expert interventions required to accurately segment anatomical or pathological structures, especially

---

F. Tilquin and P.-H. Conze—Equally contributed.

W. Bai et al. (Eds.): Patch-MI 2018, LNCS 11075, pp. 39–47, 2018.
https://doi.org/10.1007/978-3-030-00500-9_5

in pre-operative surgery planning. An alternative to avoid performing costly dense registration on highly-resolved 3D images is to reach semi-dense registration by finding correspondences between structural entities. In this context, the use of supervoxel over-segmentation techniques followed by supervoxel matching have been recently introduced [2–4]. Supervoxel over-segmentation methods such as Simple Linear Iterative Clustering (SLIC) [5] provide reliable support regions by grouping adjacent voxels into intensity-homogeneous regions. While preserving image geometry and object contours, supervoxels are able to drag dense - millions to billions of voxels - registration problems to semi-dense - thousand of supervoxels - tractable problems, bringing computational and memory gains.

This paper focuses on semi-dense pairwise supervoxel-based registration, which consists in establishing pairings between supervoxels decomposing two 3D images. Matching can be performed by aggregating voxel-wise labels within supervoxel boundaries of the second image, based on the results of a classification algorithm trained on the first image [2,3] or by direct nearest-neighbor search [4,6]. Those algorithms all depend on intensity similarity features which can be easily corrupted by uniform areas, appearance changes or different noise levels between images. Thus, the need for other multivariate and invariant representations of supervoxels arises naturally. In this paper, we focus on spectral features which have proven to be robust in dense registration problems [7].

Spectral graph methods are a variety of graph-based techniques, commonly used in dimension reduction as for Laplacian eigenmaps [8], whose goal is to find a non-linear and low-dimensional representation of high-dimensional data. Conversely, we aim at obtaining a high-dimensional supervoxel representation from 4D data arising when considering supervoxel averaged intensities and centroid positions. The spectral representation achieved at the supervoxel level relies on spectral graph decomposition followed by spectrum rearrangement. Since such features exhibit smooth spatial variations, we additionally introduce context-rich features extended from voxels [2,3,9] to supervoxels to describe the broadened spatial context on spectral representations. Accurate supervoxel correspondences are finally obtained by nearest neighbor search on these mid-level features.

Our approach is evaluated against state-of-the-art methods for semi-dense longitudinal registration of abdominal CT scans which remains an open issue due to wide organ size, shape and appearance heterogeneity.

2   Problem Formulation

Automatic semi-dense image registration is considered between two 3D images I_f and I_s. Let $\mathcal{F} = \{f_i\}_{i \in \{1,\ldots,|\mathcal{F}|\}}$ and $\mathcal{S} = \{s_j\}_{j \in \{1,\ldots,|\mathcal{S}|\}}$ be respectively the set of $|\mathcal{F}|$ and $|\mathcal{S}|$ connected supervoxels partitioning I_f and I_s and obtained using a 3D extension of SLIC [5]. Our goal is to establish supervoxel correspondences by estimating a function h that maps each supervoxel $f_i \in \mathcal{F}$ of I_f to a supervoxel $s_j \in \mathcal{S}$ of I_s, such that:

$$\forall i \in \{1,\ldots,|\mathcal{F}|\}, \exists j \in \{1,\ldots,|\mathcal{S}|\} \mid h(f_i) = s_j \tag{1}$$

We focus on supervoxel matching through straightforward nearest neighbor search at the supervoxel level. This considerably alleviates the computational and memory issues raised when a voxel-wise classification scheme [2,3] is followed. Let $\psi(f_i)$ (resp. $\psi(s_j)$) be the set of mid-level features assigned to f_i (resp. s_j). The optimization scheme can be easily written as:

$$h(f_i) = s_j = \arg\min_{s_l \in \mathcal{S}} \|\psi(f_i) - \psi(s_l)\|_2 \tag{2}$$

Since intensity-based similarity features [4,6] are not robust enough to discriminate supervoxels, alternate invariant representations of supervoxels are required. Our contributions rely on the combination of new feature categories built at the supervoxel extent: mid-level spectral and context-rich features.

3   Mid-Level Spectral Features

Spectral dimension reduction methods aim at changing the representation of high-dimensional data to a low-dimensional description with a few variables only. This embedding is expected to be as faithful to the data geometry as possible by preserving inner manifold distances in high-dimensional space, while striving to constrain the low-dimensional structure in an Euclidean space. We propose to adapt this concept in the inverse direction to provide a powerful multivariate representation of supervoxels, starting from low-dimensional 4D data arising when considering supervoxel averaged intensities and centroid positions only. In practice, we exploit for each image I_f and I_s an adjacency graph over the set of all supervoxels in order to obtain a spectral representation of chosen dimension.

3.1   Laplacian Graph Building

In the dense context [7], one usually constructs a graph where each node is a voxel and each vertex is weighted by the distance from neighboring voxels based on spatial and intensity similarities. In practice, the dense approach constrains to use only adjacency between voxels and their closest neighbors because a full matrix would be intractable from a memory and computational point of view. Conversely, we use a dense graph over the generated supervoxels. We exploit the same criteria of spatial and intensity proximity to define the adjacency graph using supervoxels as nodes and a distance between averaged positions and intensities as edges. We can thus define a dissimilarity matrix W as:

$$W_{i,j} = |X_i - X_j|/S_X + \alpha|I_i - I_j|/S_I \tag{3}$$

where i, j are indices of two supervoxels, $S_X = \sigma(\{|X_i - X_j|\}_{i,j})$ and $S_I = \sigma(\{|I_i - I_j|\}_{i,j})$ are respectively the standard deviation of differences in centroid positions and averaged intensities (X and I) of supervoxels. The balance between both terms is adjusted using α. We then define an affinity matrix A by using a Radial Basis Function (RBF) kernel over W such that: $A = \exp(-\gamma * W)$.

$\{I_f, I_s\}$ (a) without permutations and sign flips   (b) with permutations and sign flips

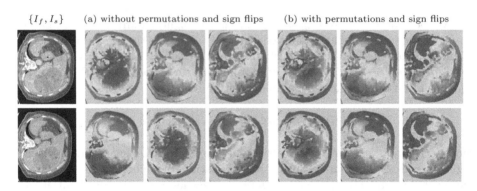

Fig. 1. First three eigenvectors with eigenvalue in increasing order without (a) and with (b) permutations and sign flips (supervoxel graphs built on two close CT scans).

The kernel introduces a non-linearity in the representation, which allows to capture the non-linear modes of intensity displacements within images. Finally, the Laplacian graph is built by performing a symmetric normalization of A:

$$L = I - D^{-1/2}AD^{-1/2} \qquad (4)$$

where I is the square identity matrix of size $|\mathcal{F}|$ for I_f or $|\mathcal{S}|$ for I_s, and D is the diagonal matrix where each diagonal coefficient corresponds to the sum of coefficients along the rows of L. By normalizing the Laplacian, we construct a Markov chain over the set of supervoxels whose eigenvectors can intuitively be interpreted as diffusion modes over the supervoxels graph.

We are now interested in computing the smallest eigenvectors of L. This can be done with any power-method based algorithm [10] for efficiency or by computing the full spectrum of L and keeping only the smallest eigenvalues. Since $|\mathcal{F}|$ and $|\mathcal{S}|$ are usually small, the computational time for the full spectrum is, in practice, in the order of a few seconds. While we lose resolution by aggregating voxels together, we consider the adjacency between all supervoxels, and not only the closest ones as imposed in dense scenarios. This allows to better capture global as well as local modes of intensity diffusion within images.

3.2   Rearrangement of the Spectra

The graph building procedure is applied to I_f and I_s. Since we compute eigenvectors of two different matrices and expect them to be similar, we should keep in mind that they are defined up to the sign and to a positive multiplicative constant. To have meaningful correspondences of eigenvectors between two Laplacian matrices, we need to ensure that they match adequately. A second problem is related to numerical issues: eigenvalues corresponding to the same diffusion modes in the two images are usually not sorted in the same way. Thus, corresponding eigenvectors between two Laplacians are defined up to a permutation.

Figure 1a presents an example of supervoxel spectral features without matching correction. We can see matching errors due to a permutation and a sign flip. To alleviate both problems, we spread the eigenvectors to $[-1, 1]$ by histogram equalization to eliminate the multiplicative problem and ensure that eigenvectors are globally discriminative. One can then either perform linear assignment with the Hungarian algorithm [11] over the joint sets of eigenvectors and their opposites or maximize the correlation in absolute value between eigenvectors, thus finding iteratively the correspondence and the sign for each one. Figure 1b shows how the Hungarian algorithm can correct these errors.

Graph decomposition and rearrangement lead to a N-dimensional feature vector $\Phi(f_i) = \{\Phi_n(f_i)\}_{n \in \{1,...,N\}}$ for each $f_i \in \mathcal{F}$ where $\Phi_n(f_i)$ is the i-th element of the n-th eigenvector built from I_f. The same representation $\Phi(s_j)$ is adopted for each $s_j \in \mathcal{S}$ based on eigenvectors generated from I_s and belonging to $\mathbb{R}^{N \times |\mathcal{S}|}$.

4   Mid-Level Context-Rich Features

The mid-level spectral representation leads to smoothly varying spatial features (Fig. 1). We thus supplement spectral features by introducing context-rich features extended from voxels [2,3,9] to supervoxels. We do not estimate mid-level context-rich features on source images [9] as usually performed but extract them on spectral features to describe their broadened spatial context.

Each supervoxel f_i of $\mathcal{F}$ is described by its barycenter $c(f_i)$ and its mid-level spectral features $\Phi_n(f_i)$. Following [4] and similarly to pixel patches, we exploit a supervoxel patch structure called superpatch. A superpatch $P_r(f_i)$ of radius r centered on f_i aggregates supervoxels $f_l \in \mathcal{F}$ such that $\|c(f_l) - c(f_i)\|_2 \leq r$. Thus, the superpatch $P_r(f_i)$ is built by considering all supervoxels located within a fixed radius r with respect to f_i and contains necessarily f_i at least. Spectral features for each superpatch can be estimated by averaging spectral features within its boundary $\Phi_n[P_r(f_i)] = \frac{1}{|P_r(f_i)|} \sum_{f_l \in P_r(f_i)} \Phi_n(f_l)$.

The superpatch concept allows a straightforward extension of context-rich features from voxels [2,3,9] to supervoxels. In particular, for each eigenvector of index $n \in \{1, ..., N\}$, we can assign M mid-level context-rich appearance features $\psi(f_i, n) = \{\psi_m(f_i, n)\}_{m \in \{0,...,M\}}$ to each supervoxel f_i following:

$$\psi_m(f_i, n) = \Phi_n[P_r(\mathcal{N}_\Delta(f_i))] - b \times \Phi_n[P_{r'}(\mathcal{N}_{\Delta'}(f_i))] \tag{5}$$

where $\mathcal{N}_\Delta(f_i)$ defines an extended supervoxel neighbor of f_i reached by applying displacement Δ starting from barycenter $c(f_i)$. Thus, $\mathcal{N}_\Delta(f_i)$ corresponds to the supervoxel containing location $c(f_i) + \Delta$. Displacements $\{\Delta, \Delta'\}$ are randomly defined in a ball of maximal radius ε. Radii $\{r, r'\}$ are computed following $r = q \times \frac{\kappa}{2}$ where κ is an averaged inter-barycenter distance (estimated among all adjacent supervoxels) and q designates an integer randomly generated within $\{1, 2, ..., Q\}$. $b \in \{0, 1\}$ is a binary parameter which selects whether the average spectral feature differences between two superpatches randomly located in the extended neighborhood of f_i ($b = 1$) or the value obtained from one single superpatch

$P_r(\mathcal{N}_\Delta(f_i))$ only $(b = 0)$. Averaged spectral features around f_i are included in the feature vector $\psi(f_i, n)$ by forcing $\Delta = b = 0$ for all possible radii r.

By randomly generating many different radii r and offsets Δ, we obtain M features describing the extended spatial context at a mid-level extend for spectral representations corresponding to the n-th eigenvalue. For each eigenvalue, $\{\Delta, \Delta', r, r', b\}$ are randomly generated once and remain similar for each supervoxel and each image. Conversely, these parameters differ from one eigenvalue to another. The combination of spectral and context-rich features leads to $N \times M$ features $\psi(\cdot) = [\psi(\cdot, 1), \psi(\cdot, 2), ..., \psi(\cdot, N)] \in \mathbb{R}^{N \times M}$ assigned to each supervoxel.

5   Results

Experiments focus on data collected from 45 images pairs from 18 examinations, stemming from 7 patients with hepato-cellular carcinoma. Each pair brings together two dynamic contrast-enhanced (DCE-)CT scans acquired for the same patient and the same phase (before injection, arterial, early venous or late venous), at different time points varying from 41 to 700 days (226 in average). Image pairs are processed both forward (FW) and backward (BW) to get mapping functions $h_{\text{FW}}(f_i) = s_j$ and $h_{\text{BW}}(s_j) = f_i$ for each supervoxel $f_i \in \mathcal{F}$ and $s_j \in \mathcal{S}$.

Since supervoxel matching allows a straightforward propagation of anatomical labels, we evaluate the proposed methodology on liver label propagation results using DICE scores comparing liver propagation and ground-truth (GT) masks. Supervoxel pairings are also assessed using FW/BW inconsistency scores defined for each supervoxel similarly to $\text{inc}(f_i) = \|c(f_i) - c(h_{\text{BW}}(h_{\text{FW}}(f_i)))\|_2$.

The dataset is used to compare the proposed supervoxel matching combining mid-level spectral and context-rich features (sm-SC) with baseline techniques including supervoxel matching through mid-level intensity histogram (sm-I), spectral (sm-S) and intensity-based context-rich features (sm-IC) only, state-of-the-art SuperPatchMatch [4] (spm-I) and unsupervised learning-based voxel-to-supervoxel mapping using pixel-wise intensity-based context-rich features [2] (uvm-C). Supervoxel pairings for sm-{I,S,IC,SC} are established through nearest neighbor search contrary to uvm-C which employs voxel-wise random forests (RF) [12]. sm-I and spm-I use 30 bins intensity histograms. Strategies based on spectral features (sm-{S,SC}) use $N = 17$ eigenvectors. The total feature number for sm-{C,SC} and uvm-C is 600 (595 for sm-SC with $N = 17$ and $M = 35$). Affinity matrices for sm-SC are computed with $\alpha = 0.1$ (Eq. 3) and $\gamma = 0.1$. Superpatch radii are estimated with $Q = 4$ for sm-SC and $r = \frac{3 \times \kappa}{2}$ for spm-I (Sect. 4) whereas averaged intensities for usm-C are considered with box sizes $\{3,5,7,9\}$. spm-I employs 6 iterations including propagation and random search. The maximal ball radius used to define extended neighbors for $\{\text{sm-SC}, \text{usm-C}\}$ is $\varepsilon = 125$.

Partitions are made of $|\mathcal{F}| = |\mathcal{S}| = 2000$ supervoxels defined within areas with intensities in the $[-200, 200]$ Hounsfield unit range. A SLIC [5] compactness of 0.2 with intensities rescaled to $[0, 1]$ reaches a good trade-off between compactness and boundary adherence. Methods are applied with two SLIC decompositions: without and with a-priori liver segmentation awareness to evaluate supervoxel matches without being disturbed by boundary adherence issues. With a-priori, decompositions are separately performed for liver and other abdominal structures depending on relative volumes and merged to obtain one single partition.

Table 1. Quantitative comparisons of the proposed supervoxel matching combining mid-level spectral and context-rich features (`sm-SC`) with baseline techniques (`sm-I`, `sm-S`, `sm-IC`, `spm-I` [4], `uvm-C` [2]) through liver label propagation (`DICE`) and inconsistency (`inc`) averaged over the database (`FW` and `BW`). Best results are in bold.

SLIC	Metric	sm-I	sm-IC	sm-S	spm-I [4]	uvm-C [2]	sm-SC (ours)
no a-priori	DICE	58.87	77.84 ± 0.10	83.26	66.85 ± 1.78	81.83 ± 0.12	$\mathbf{86.28 \pm 0.06}$
	inc	27.56	10.71 ± 0.05	8.01	50.19 ± 1.05	15.89 ± 0.09	$\mathbf{7.46 \pm 0.05}$
a-priori	DICE	60.49	78.89 ± 0.28	80.31	70.52 ± 1.07	80.71 ± 0.13	$\mathbf{87.02 \pm 0.10}$
	inc	27.14	10.74 ± 0.05	8.57	51.67 ± 2.03	16.20 ± 0.10	$\mathbf{7.70 \pm 0.06}$

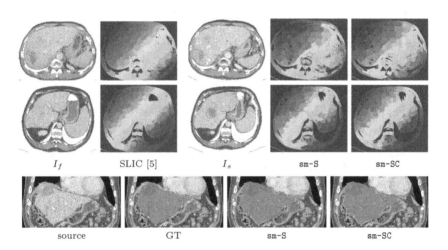

I_f SLIC [5] I_s sm-S   sm-SC

source   GT   sm-S   sm-SC

Fig. 2. Assessment of `sm-{S,SC}` with supervoxel decomposition and pairings, GT and propagated liver mask (without a-priori).

Average `DICE` and `inc` scores, displayed in Table 1, demonstrate that `sm-SC` achieves the highest segmentation accuracy along with the lowest inconsistency in both configurations. Without liver segmentation awareness, significant gains in `DICE` (`inc`) arise with 86.28 (7.46) against 83.26 (8.01) and 81.83 (15.89) for `sm-S` and `uvm-C` respectively. More substantial gains arise using a-priori with `DICE` improvements of 6.7 (6.3) with respect to `sm-S` (`uvm-C`). `sm-{S,SC}` outperforms `uvm-C` whose computational and memory requirements are much higher since voxel-wise RF are used. Results show that intensity features (`{sm-I,spm-I}`) are not robust enough to discriminate supervoxels without context-rich or spectral descriptions. Compared to sm-S, applying context-rich features on spectral representations (sm-SC) reaches gains around 6.7 (3.0) and 0.9 (0.55) in DICE and inc with (without) a-priori. Comparing sm-IC and sm-SC reveals that context-rich features are more efficient on spectral than CT intensity data. The significant impact of the newly designed mid-level features are highlighted in Fig. 2 illustrating the accuracy of both supervoxel matching and liver propagation.

6   Conclusion

This work addresses automatic semi-dense image registration relying on robust supervoxel matching. We propose new multivariate supervoxel representations embedded in nearest neighbor search. Feature extraction is performed at the supervoxel level and combines mid-level spectral and context-rich information. Spectral graph decomposition and spectrum rearrangement are involved to capture global modes of intensity diffusion within supervoxel adjacency graphs. Context-rich features extended from voxels to supervoxels are employed to describe the extended spatial context on resulting spectral representations. Experiments on liver label propagation between CT image pairs show that our strategy outperforms state-of-the-art methods while bringing computational and memory gains. Extending this work to multi-scale supervoxel decomposition would deserve further investigation to drive the matching process in a coarse-to-fine fashion. This work also gives new insights for registration initialization, towards more complex dense deformation model estimation. Finally, we plan to explore spectral supervoxel matching for multi-phases and multi-modal registration.

Acknowledgments. This work was partly funded by France Life Imaging (grant ANR-11-INBS-0006 from Investissements d'Avenir program). We acknowledge Visible Patient, www.visiblepatient.com, for 3D liver segmentation masks.

References

1. Schnabel, J.A., Heinrich, M.P., Papież, B.W., Brady, J.M.: Advances and challenges in deformable image registration: from image fusion to complex motion modelling. Med. Image Anal. **33**, 145–148 (2016)
2. Kanavati, F., Tong, T., Misawa, K., Fujiwara, M., Mori, K., Rueckert, D., Glocker, B.: Supervoxel classification forests for estimating pairwise image correspondences. Pattern Recogn. **63**, 561–569 (2017)
3. Conze, P.H., Tilquin, F., Noblet, V., Rousseau, F., Heitz, F., Pessaux, P.: Hierarchical multi-scale supervoxel matching using random forests for automatic semi-dense abdominal image registration. In: International Symposium on Biomedical Imaging (2017)
4. Giraud, R., Ta, V.T., Bugeau, A., Coupé, P., Papadakis, N.: Superpatchmatch: an algorithm for robust correspondences using superpixel patches. IEEE Trans. Image Process. **26**(8), 4068–4078 (2017)

5. Achanta, R., Shaji, A., Smith, K., Lucchi, A., Fua, P., Susstrunk, S.: SLIC super-pixels compared to state-of-the-art superpixel methods. IEEE Trans. Pattern Anal. Mach. Intell. **34**(11), 2274–2282 (2012)
6. Fan, H., Xiang, J., Chen, Z.: Visual tracking by local superpixel matching with Markov random field. In: Pacific Rim Conference on Multimedia (2016)
7. Lombaert, H., Grady, L., Pennec, X., Ayache, N., Cheriet, F.: Spectral log-demons: diffeomorphic image registration with very large deformations. Int. J. Comput. Vis. **107**(3), 254–271 (2014)
8. Belkin, M., Niyogi, P.: Laplacian Eigenmaps and spectral techniques for embedding and clustering. In: Advances in Neural Information Processing Systems (2002)
9. Criminisi, A., Shotton, J., Robertson, D., Konukoglu, E.: Regression forests for efficient anatomy detection and localization in CT studies. In: MICCAI Workshop on Medical Computer Vision, pp. 106–117 (2010)
10. Arnoldi, W.E.: The principle of minimized iterations in the solution of the matrix eigenvalue problem. Q. Appl. Math. **9**(1), 17–29 (1951)
11. Kuhn, H.W.: The Hungarian method for the assignment problem. Naval Res. Logist. **2**, 83–97 (1955)
12. Breiman, L.: Random forests. Mach. Learn. **45**(1), 5–32 (2001)

Stereo Matching for Wireless Capsule Endoscopy Using Direct Attenuation Model

Min-Gyu Park[✉], Ju Hong Yoon, and Youngbae Hwang

Intelligent Image Processing Research Center, Korea Electronics Technology Institute (KETI), Gwangju, South Korea
{mpark,jhyoon,ybhwang}@keti.re.kr

Abstract. We propose a robust approach to estimate depth maps designed for stereo camera-based wireless capsule endoscopy. Since there is no external light source except ones attached to the capsule, we employ the direct attenuation model to estimate a depth map up to a scale factor. Afterward, we estimate the scale factor by using sparse feature correspondences. Finally, the estimated depth map is used to guide stereo matching to recover the detailed structure of the captured scene. We experimentally verify the proposed method with various images captured by stereo-type endoscopic capsules in the gastrointestinal tract.

1 Introduction

The wireless capsule endoscope (WCE) is a powerful device to acquire images of the gastrointestinal (GI) tract for screening, diagnostic, and therapeutic endoscopic procedures [1]. Especially, the WCE captures the images of the small intestine where current wired endoscopic devices cannot reach. In this paper, we introduce a method to recover the 3D structure from stereo images captured by a stereo-type WCE, shown in Fig. 1.

To perceive depth from endoscopic images, many researchers have brought various computer vision techniques such as stereo matching [4], shape-from-shading (SfS) [2,13], shape-from-focus (SfF) [11], and shape-from-motion (SfM) [3]. Ciuti et al. [2] adopted the SfS technique because the position of light sources are known and shading is an important cue in the endoscopic images. Visentini et al. [13] fused the SfS cue and image feature correspondences to estimate accurate dense disparity maps. Takeshita et al. [11] introduced an endoscopic device that estimates depth by using the SfF technique, which utilizes multiple images captured with different focus settings at the same camera position. Fan et al. [3] established sparse feature correspondences between consequent images, and then, they calculated camera poses and the 3D structure of the scene by using the SfM technique. They generated 3D meshes through Delaunay triangulation by using triangulated feature points.

Stereo matching is also a well-known technique to estimate a depth map from images, which can be divided into active and passive [9] approaches. We refer

© Springer Nature Switzerland AG 2018
W. Bai et al. (Eds.): Patch-MI 2018, LNCS 11075, pp. 48–56, 2018.
https://doi.org/10.1007/978-3-030-00500-9_6

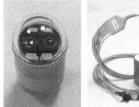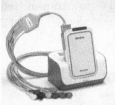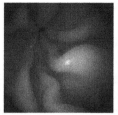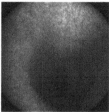

Fig. 1. Stereo-type wireless endoscopic capsule, wireless receiver, and captured images in the stomach and the small bowel, from the left.

structured light-based stereo matching [10] to the active approach which projects a visible or IR pattern to the scene to leverage correspondence searching between the images. However, the active approach is not suitable for wireless endoscopy mainly because of the limited resources, e.g., battery capacity and the size of a capsule. Therefore, previous studies [4] focused on minimally invasive surgery rather than WCE-based GI examination. For the same reason, most commercial wireless endoscopic capsules typically adopt conventional passive image sensors.

To the best of our knowledge, commercially available WCE products are not capable of estimating depth information. This is the first attempt to estimate the geometric structure of the scene inside the GI tract captured by a WCE. To achieve this goal, we designed a stereo-type WCE as shown in Fig. 1 without enlarging the diameter of the capsule. This sensor can capture about 0.12 million images for the entire GI tract as described in Fig. 1 ranging from the stomach to the large bowel. Having captured stereo images in one hand, we estimate a fully dense depth map by using the direct attenuation model. Since there is no external light source except ones attached to the capsule, farther objects look darker than nearer one in the captured image. Therefore, we consider the attenuation trend of the light to estimate depth maps assuming that the medium inside the GI tract is homogeneous. We firstly employ the direct attenuation model to compute an up-to-scale depth map, and then, solve the scale ambiguity by using sparse feature correspondences. Afterward, we utilize the rescaled depth map to guide a popularly used algorithm, i.e., semi-global matching (SGM) [6]. The detailed description of the proposed method is given in the following section.

2 Proposed Method

2.1 Capsule Specification

Our wireless endoscopic capsule consists of two cameras, four led lights, a wireless transmitter, and the battery. Two cameras are displaced about 4 mm, the viewing angle is 170°, and the resolution of captured images is 320 × 320. The capsule captures three pairs of images per second. In total, it captures more than 115,000 images for eight hours in the GI tract. Four led lights are attached around the cameras as shown in Fig. 1. The lights are synchronized with the cameras to minimize the battery usage. Captured images are transmitted to the receiver because the capsule does not have an internal storage. The length of the capsule is 24 mm and the diameter is 11 mm.

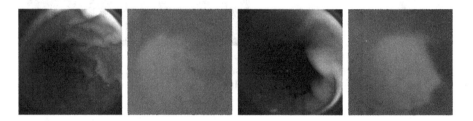

Fig. 2. Sample input images and the depth maps computed by Eq. (5). Here, bright pixels indicates they are farther than dark ones.

2.2　Depth Estimation with the Direct Attenuation Model

Since the captured image has poor visibility, the image for each pixel $\mathbf{p}$ can be modeled as [5]

$$I(\mathbf{p}) = J(\mathbf{p})t(\mathbf{p}) + A(1 - t(\mathbf{p})), \tag{1}$$

where J is the scene radiance, I is the observed intensity, t is the transmission map, and A is the atmospheric light. Since there is no source of natural illumination such as sunlight, A can be dropped from Eq. (1). Then, t can be defined as

$$t(\mathbf{p}) = I(\mathbf{p})/J(\mathbf{p}). \tag{2}$$

The transmission map also can be defined by Bouguer's exponential law of attenuation [8],

$$t(\mathbf{p}) = \exp\left(-\beta(\mathbf{p})d(\mathbf{p})\right), \tag{3}$$

where an attenuation coefficient $\beta(\mathbf{p})$ is typically represented by sum of absorption and scattering coefficients, $\beta(\mathbf{p}) = \beta_{\text{absortion}}(\mathbf{p}) + \beta_{\text{scatter}}(\mathbf{p})$. By combining Eqs. (2) and (3), the depth of a pixel $\mathbf{p}$ can be estimated as

$$d(\mathbf{p}) = \frac{\ln(J(\mathbf{p})) - \ln(I(\mathbf{p}))}{\beta(\mathbf{p})} \approx \frac{\ln(\bar{I}) - \ln(I(\mathbf{p}))}{\beta}. \tag{4}$$

To simplify Eq.(4), we approximate two terms $J(\mathbf{p})$ and $\beta(\mathbf{p})$ by considering characteristics of the GI tract. First, assuming that the GI tract is filled with a homogeneous matter such as water, the attenuation coefficient $\beta(\mathbf{p})$ is approximated as a constant value for all pixels, $\beta \approx \beta(\mathbf{p})$. Second, we also approximate the scene radiance as the mean of all pixel values as $J(\mathbf{p}) \approx \bar{I}$ based on the assumption that most pixels have a similar color in a local GI region. Based on the second assumption, we easily obtain the depth map up to a scale factor β,

$$d_\beta(\mathbf{p}) = \beta\, d(\mathbf{p}) = \ln(\bar{I}) - \ln(I(\mathbf{p})). \tag{5}$$

Here, the depth map $d_\beta(\mathbf{p})$ indicates a depth map up to scale factor β. In the following section, we estimate β. Beforehand, we apply a noise removal filter to smooth $d_\beta(\mathbf{p})$ by using a well-known bilateral filter [12].

2.3 Resolving the Scale Ambiguity of d_β

To resolve the scale ambiguity of $d_\beta(\mathbf{p})$, we compute β from by using sparse feature correspondences. First, we detect and match corner points. Then, we compute the depth of $\mathbf{p}$, $d_s(\mathbf{p})$,

$$d_s(\mathbf{p}) = \frac{fB}{|p_x^L - p_x^R|}, \tag{6}$$

where p_x^L and p_x^R are the positions of matched points from the left and right images along the x-axis, f is the focal length of the left camera, B is the baseline between two cameras. Since each corner point has corresponding $d_\beta(\mathbf{p})$, β can be computed by

$$\beta = d_\beta(\mathbf{p})/d_s(\mathbf{p}). \tag{7}$$

Assuming that β is constant for all pixels, we find an optimal β, β^*, that maximizes the number of inlier points whose error is smaller than a threshold value, τ_c.

$$\beta^* = \arg\max_{\beta \in \mathcal{B}} \sum_{\mathbf{p} \in \mathcal{S}} T(\mathbf{p}, \beta, \tau_c),$$
$$T(\mathbf{p}, \beta, \tau_c) = \begin{cases} 1 \text{ if } |d_s(\mathbf{p}) - d_\beta(\mathbf{p})/\beta| \leq \tau_c \\ 0 \qquad\qquad \text{otherwise.} \end{cases}, \tag{8}$$

where $\mathcal{B}$ is the set of β values computed from all feature correspondences and $\mathcal{S}$ is the set of correspondences' positions in the image coordinate. The function T gives 1, if the discrepancy between $d_s(\mathbf{p})$ and rescaled $d_\beta(\mathbf{p})$ is small, and 0, otherwise. Therefore, the estimated β^* minimizes the gap between d_s and d_β/β. We thus rescale $d_\beta(\mathbf{p})$ and compute its corresponding disparity map as

$$\bar{d}_\beta(\mathbf{p}) = \frac{d_\beta(\mathbf{p})}{\beta^*}, \quad \bar{D}_\beta(\mathbf{p}) = \frac{fB}{\bar{d}_\beta(\mathbf{p})}. \tag{9}$$

We utilize the rescaled disparity map $\bar{D}_\beta(\mathbf{p})$ to leverage stereo matching.

2.4 Robust Stereo Matching Using a Guidance Depth Map

We slightly modify the SGM algorithm [6] to compute the disparity map $D(\mathbf{p})$ which minimizes the following energy function,

$$E(d) = \sum_{\mathbf{p}} (\phi(\mathbf{p}, D(\mathbf{p})) + \psi(\mathbf{p}, D(\mathbf{p})))$$
$$+ \sum_{\mathbf{q} \in N_\mathbf{p}} P_1 T[|D(\mathbf{p}) - D(\mathbf{q})| = 1] + \sum_{\mathbf{q} \in N_\mathbf{p}} P_2 T[|D(\mathbf{p}) - D(\mathbf{q})| > 1]. \tag{10}$$

In the first term, the function $\phi(\cdot, \cdot)$ is the pixel-wise matching cost, computed by using Census-based hamming distance and absolute difference of intensities (AD-CENSUS). The function $\psi(\cdot, \cdot)$ is also the pixel-wise matching cost computed by using $\bar{D}_\beta(\mathbf{p})$,

$$\psi(\mathbf{p}, D(\mathbf{p})) = \begin{cases} |\bar{D}_\beta(\mathbf{p}) - D(\mathbf{p})| & \text{if } |\bar{D}_\beta(\mathbf{p}) - D(\mathbf{p})| \leq \tau_{\text{err}} \\ c & \text{otherwise} \end{cases}. \qquad (11)$$

The second term gives the penalty P_1 for the pixels having small disparity differences with the neighboring pixels $\mathbf{q} \in N_\mathbf{p}$, i.e., $T[|D(\mathbf{p}) - D(\mathbf{q})| = 1]$ gives 1 when the difference of disparity values is 1. Similarly, the third term gives the large penalty P_2 such that $P_2 > P_1$ for the pixels having disparity differences greater than 1 with the neighboring pixels. We minimize Eq. 10 by using the SGM method [6]. As a post-processing step, we apply the weighted median filter [7]. Finally, we obtain the depth map from the disparity map by $d(\mathbf{p}) = fB/D(\mathbf{p})$.

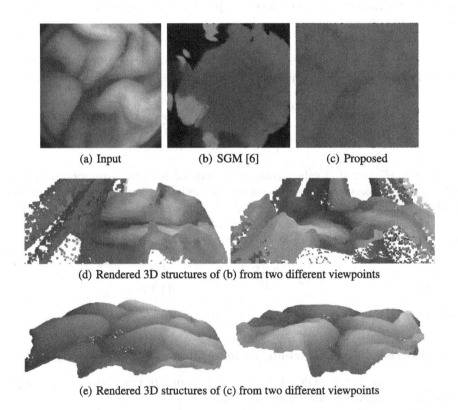

(a) Input   (b) SGM [6]   (c) Proposed

(d) Rendered 3D structures of (b) from two different viewpoints

(e) Rendered 3D structures of (c) from two different viewpoints

Fig. 3. Comparison of disparity maps and reconstructed 3D structures.

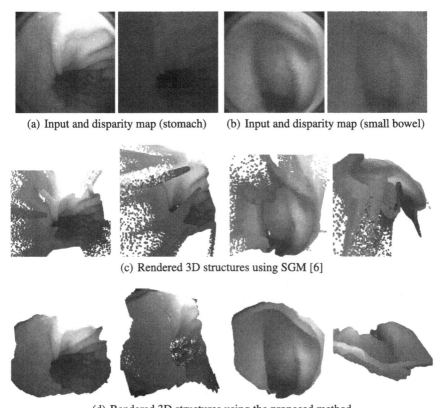

(a) Input and disparity map (stomach)   (b) Input and disparity map (small bowel)

(c) Rendered 3D structures using SGM [6]

(d) Rendered 3D structures using the proposed method

Fig. 4. Comparison reconstructed 3D structures.

3 Experimental Results

Computing depth maps from endoscopic images is difficult, mainly because of difficulties caused by the characteristics of the GI tract and the limited resources of the capsule. The difficulties are summarized as (1) inaccurate matching due to lens distortion, (2) low resolution image, (3) image noise caused by the lack of illumination.

Note that the proposed method without the direct attenuation model and its cost function terms in Eqs. (10) and (11) is identical to the popularly used stereo matching algorithm, SGM [6]. Therefore, we qualitatively compare results of the proposed method with the conventional SGM to demonstrate the advantages of the proposed method under the aforementioned difficulties. To achieve fair comparison and to explicitly demonstrate the advantages of the proposed method, we used the same similarity measure and parameters for the SGM and the proposed method.

In the first experiment, we used the images of a stomach and a small bowel captured by our stereo-type WCE. In the second experiment, we used the large bowel Phantom model[1] not only to capture endoscopic images but also to compare the actual size of an object with the estimated size.

Qualitative Evaluation: Most importantly, the proposed method acquires fully dense depth maps whereas the conventional approach fails at non-overlapping regions because pixels of the left image in non-overlapping regions do not have corresponding pixels of the right image. Moreover, since we used a large field of view cameras, the proportion of non-overlapping regions is about 30~50% depending on the distance of the captured scene from the camera. Computed disparity values in non-overlapping regions are noisy as shown in Fig. 3(b) where noisy disparity values are exceptionally brighter than others in the disparity map although they should show similar disparity as seen in the scene structure of Fig. 3(a). The noisy disparity values become more conspicuous when they are represented in the 3D space as shown in Fig. 3(d), and those noisy disparity values seem to float the space so that they obstruct to see the underlying 3D structure. Differently, the proposed method accurately recovers the 3D structure of the scene as shown in Fig. 3(e) because the proposed cost function with the direct attenuation model well suppresses uncertainties caused by radial distortion and low light noise. In addition, the depth map based on the direct attenuation model effectively enforces the proposed cost function to reconstruct the depth in non-overlapping regions as shown in Fig. 3(c).

As discussed in the introduction, the main advantage of the WCE is that it can capture not only stomach images but also images of small bowel where typical wired endoscopic devices cannot reach. Similar to the results demonstrated in Fig. 3, the proposed method reconstruct 3D structures of the local stomach and small bowel regions more robustly than the SGM as shown in Figs. 4(c) and (d), and effectively estimates dense depth maps in non-overlapping regions as shown in Figs. 4(a) and (b).

Application for Diagnosis: We also show an application of the proposed method for diagnosis. Using estimated depth information, we estimate the size of an object of interest by clicking two points from the image as shown in Figs. 5(a) and (c). In this experiment, we used the large bowel Phantom model and two different types of polyps whose size is known. As shown in Figs. 5, the estimated size is quite similar to the actual size in which the error was at most 0.5 mm. This procedure has long relied on the experienced doctor or endoscopist.

Parameter Settings and Running Time: We used 7×9 window to compute census-based matching cost computation, and set P1 and P2 to 11 and 19, respectively. The average running time of the proposed method was about 10ms, implemented on a modern GPU, GTX Titan Xp.

---

[1] https://www.buyamag.com/digestive_system_models.php.

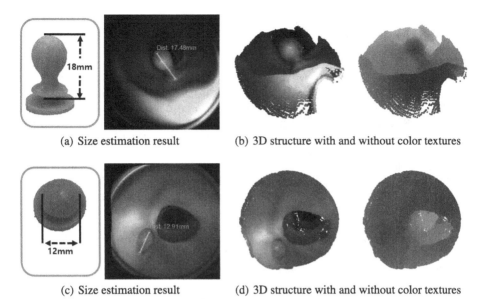

(a) Size estimation result   (b) 3D structure with and without color textures

(c) Size estimation result   (d) 3D structure with and without color textures

Fig. 5. Size estimation results with a large bowel Phantom model

4   Conclusion

We have proposed a stereo matching algorithm designed for a stereo-type wire-less capsule endoscopy. We obtained an up-to-scale depth map by using the direct attenuation model because of the light source around the capsule in the completely dark environment. Thereafter, we employed the up-to-scale depth map to guide conventional stereo matching algorithms after resolving the scale ambiguity. Through the experiments, we observed that the proposed method can estimate depth maps accurately and robustly in the GI tract.

Acknowledgment. This work was supported by 'The Cross-Ministry Giga KOREA Project' grant funded by the Korea government(MSIT) (No. K18P0200, Development of 4D reconstruction and dynamic deformable action model based hyper-realistic service technology) and a gift from Intromedic.

References

1. Ciuti, G., Menciassi, A., Dario, P.: Capsule endoscopy: from current achievements to open challenges. IEEE Rev. Biomed. Eng. **4**, 59–72 (2011)
2. Ciuti, G., Visentini-Scarzanella, M., Dore, A., Menciassi, A., Dario, P., Yang, G.Z.: Intra-operative monocular 3d reconstruction for image-guided navigation in active locomotion capsule endoscopy. In: 2012 4th IEEE RAS EMBS International Conference on Biomedical Robotics and Biomechatronics (BioRob), pp. 768–774, June 2012

3. Fan, Y., Meng, M.Q.H., Li, B.: 3d reconstruction of wireless capsule endoscopy images. In: 2010 Annual International Conference of the IEEE Engineering in Medicine and Biology, pp. 5149–5152, August 2010

4. Furukawa, R., Sanomura, Y., Tanaka, S., Yoshida, S., Sagawa, R., Visentini-Scarzanella, M., Kawasaki, H.: 3d endoscope system using doe projector. In: 2016 38th Annual International Conference of the IEEE Engineering in Medicine and Biology Society (EMBC), pp. 2091–2094, August 2016

5. He, K., Sun, J., Tang, X.: Single image haze removal using dark channel prior. IEEE Trans. Pattern Anal. Mach. Intell. 33(12), 2341–2353 (2011). https://doi.org/10.1109/TPAMI.2010.168

6. Hirschmüller, H.: Stereo processing by semiglobal matching and mutual information. IEEE Trans. Pattern Anal. Mach. Intell. 30(2), 328–341 (2008)

7. Ma, Z., He, K., Wei, Y., Sun, J., Wu, E.: Constant time weighted median filtering for stereo matching and beyond. In: IEEE International Conference on Computer Vision (ICCV) (2013)

8. Narasimhan, S.G., Nayar, S.K.: Vision and the atmosphere. Int. J. Comput. Vis. 48(3), 233–254 (2002). https://doi.org/10.1023/A:1016328200723

9. Scharstein, D., Szeliski, R.: A taxonomy and evaluation of dense two-frame stereo correspondence algorithms. Int. J. Comput. Vis. 47, 7–42 (2002)

10. Scharstein, D., Szeliski, R.: High-accuracy stereo depth maps using structured light. In: Proceedings of the 2003 IEEE Computer Society Conference on Computer Vision and Pattern Recognition, CVPR 2003, pp. 195–202. IEEE Computer Society, Washington, DC, USA (2003). http://dl.acm.org/citation.cfm?id=1965841.1965865

11. Takeshita, T., Kim, M., Nakajima, Y.: 3-d shape measurement endoscope using a single-lens system. Int. J. Comput. Assist. Radiol. Surg. 8(3), 451–459 (2013). https://doi.org/10.1007/s11548-012-0794-2

12. Tomasi, C., Manduchi, R.: Bilateral filtering for gray and color images. In: IEEE International Conference on Computer Vision (ICCV) (1998)

13. Visentini-Scarzanella, M., Stoyanov, D.: Stereo and shape-from-shading cue fusion for dense 3d reconstruction in endoscopic surgery. In: 3rd Joint Workshop on New Technologies for Computer/Robot Assisted Surgery (CRAS) (2013). https://drive.google.com/open?id=0B0x0v_kN6YuManhfYXVtSjJDYnc

Image Classification and Detection

Liver Tissue Classification Using an Auto-context-based Deep Neural Network with a Multi-phase Training Framework

Fan Zhang[1]($\boxtimes$), Junlin Yang[1], Nariman Nezami[3], Fabian Laage-gaupp[3],
Julius Chapiro[3], Ming De Lin[3,4], and James Duncan[1,2]

[1] Department of Biomedical Engineering, Yale University, New Haven, CT, USA
fan.zhang@yale.edu
[2] Department of Electrical Engineering, Yale University,
New Haven, CT, USA
[3] Department of Radiology and Biomedical Imaging, Yale University,
New Haven, CT, USA
[4] Philips Research North America, Cambridge, MA, USA

Abstract. In this project, our goal is to classify different types of liver tissue on 3D multi-parameter magnetic resonance images in patients with hepatocellular carcinoma. In these cases, 3D fully annotated segmentation masks from experts are expensive to acquire, thus the dataset available for training a predictive model is usually small. To achieve the goal, we designed a novel deep convolutional neural network that incorporates auto-context elements directly into a U-net-like architecture. We used a patch-based strategy with a weighted sampling procedure in order to train on a sufficient number of samples. Furthermore, we designed a multi-resolution and multi-phase training framework to reduce the learning space and to increase the regularization of the model. Our method was tested on images from 20 patients and yielded promising results, outperforming standard neural network approaches as well as a benchmark method for liver tissue classification.

Keywords: Tissue classification · Convolutional neural network
Auto-context · Multi-phase training · Hepatocellular carcinoma
Magnetic resonance imaging

1 Introduction

Hepatocellular carcinoma (HCC) is one of the most common cancer types and the leading cause in cancer-related death [4]. Multi-parameter dynamic contrast enhanced (DCE) magnetic resonance (MR) images are commonly used as a diagnostic tool for suspected HCC cases and are important for defining treatment targets and predicting outcomes for a number of therapeutic strategies including transarterial chemoembolization (TACE) [3]. In this work, we are interested in classifying liver tissue into clinically relevant types on 3D MR images:

© Springer Nature Switzerland AG 2018
W. Bai et al. (Eds.): Patch-MI 2018, LNCS 11075, pp. 59–66, 2018.
https://doi.org/10.1007/978-3-030-00500-9_7

parenchyma and anomalies that consist of viable tumor tissue and necrosis tissue. Recent developments in the design of deep convolutional neural networks (CNN) provide ways to construct powerful models that can extract both low and high level features from images that are usually difficult to formulate with traditional methods and draw accurate inferences [5]. However, such models typically need a large amount of expert curated labels. This is particularly expensive in our case as the training requires 3D fully annotated segmentation masks from radiologists.

To overcome these challenges, we designed a novel CNN model that incorporates contextual information to perform classification in a local patch region. The input patches were sampled at a fixed size but with different resolutions, in order to capture information from different scales efficiently. We developed an auto-context-based multi-level architecture that, when coupled with a multi-phase training procedure, can effectively learn and predict at different levels. The learning space needed for the each level of the model was thus reduced, since it only needed to learn the incremental difference based on the learner in the previous level.

Several other works have explored the similar idea of combining CNN and auto-context [6,9]. Here we want to point out the difference. In a popular study [6], auto-context is applied outside the classifier to refine classification performance. Our algorithm, in contrast, applies auto-context within the multi-level classifier, efficiently integrating contextual information from multi-resolution patch samples to address the small dataset problem.

The main contributions of this work are threefold: (1) It is the first deep neural network approach to segment tissue types on multi-parameter MR images in HCC patients without the need of manually designing image features [7]. While deep CNNs have been developed for liver tumor segmentation from CT images [1,2], such approaches have not been applied to MR images. (2) It incorporates a novel auto-context based CNN model design combined with a multi-phase training strategy that encourages the model to utilize contextual information from the previous phase. This hierarchical combination of several predictive units is shown to out-perform the use of a single U-net model given the available data pool without overfitting. (3) It creatively addresses the data deficiency problem by sampling the image at different resolutions under a patch based learning scheme. These multi-resolution patches effectively integrate image information from different scales yet maintain a relatively low input dimensionality. Overall, we see the methodology employed in this work as being generalizable to a number of other detection and segmentation tasks in biomedical images where full image annotation is difficult to acquire.

2   Proposed Method

2.1   Data Preprocessing

We adopted a patch-based learning scheme in our study to address the data deficiency problem, as the model would only need to learn the probability distri-

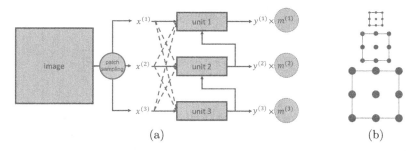

(a)   (b)

Fig. 1. Overall structure. Subfigure (a) illustrates the overall architecture of the model. $x^{(k)}$'s are the patches sampled from the image at resolution k's, $y^{(k)}$'s are the corresponding output of each unit k. $m^{(k)}$'s are different sizes of Gaussian-shape masks applied to $y^{(k)}$'s to emphasize prediction performance at the center of patches. Dashed lines between $x^{(k)}$'s and the units means connections are optional. Subfigure (b) illustrates the sampling patterns at different resolutions: the same window dimension, but different voxel-to-voxel distance

bution of each voxel at a local patch region. In addition, we designed a weighted sampling procedure to address the class imbalance problem. On average, anomalies account for only 10% of the total liver tissue. We thus re-balanced the class by forcing a sampling frequency of 50% parenchyma and 50% anomalies.

We also implemented a novel multi-resolution sampling procedure to incorporate image information at different scales in each patch. This is useful for detecting and delineating anomalies at different sizes (Fig. 1a). This multi-resolution sampling method has two advantages over simply expanding the patch size with a fixed resolution. First, the fixed patch size is more convenient to work with in CNNs. Second, the number of voxels in the input array is greatly reduced to improve computation efficiency.

To further handle the small dataset problem, we used data augmentation. Each time a patch was sampled, a 3D random rotation was applied.

2.2 Multi-level Hierarchical Architecture

The architecture we proposed is illustrated in Fig. 1b. The whole model consists of three basic units. In general, each unit k can be any CNN that outputs a probability map, but in this study we adopted the U-net architecture due to its elegant design and powerful performance [5]. The entire model took in image patches sampled at different resolutions and output predictions at those resolutions. The connection from output y^k from each unit to its higher level unit draws inspiration from the research in auto-context [8].

We used a weighted cross entropy as our loss function to update the weights in the neural network (Eq. 1), and a weighted dice similarity coefficient to monitor the training process and to select the best model (Eq. 2).

$$loss = -\sum_{x}\sum_{i} m(x)\omega(i)p(x,i)\log(q(x,i)) \tag{1}$$

$$\Omega_{h,i}(x) = 1_{\underset{j}{\mathrm{argmax}}\, h(x,j)=i}$$

$$metric_i = \frac{2\sum_x m(x)\Omega_{p,i}(x)\Omega_{q,i}(x)}{\sum_x m(x)\Omega_{p,i}(x) + \sum_x m(x)\Omega_{q,i}(x)} \qquad (2)$$

$$metric = \sum_i \alpha_i \cdot metric_i$$

In Eqs. (1) and (2), x is the location inside the patch, i is the class, p is the true probability distribution, taking only values of 0 or 1, q is the predicted probability distribution, m is a Gaussian shape mask to emphasize the performance at the center of the patch, ω and α are the weights in the loss function and the metric that are set to accentuate performance on certain classes, and $\Omega_{h,i}$ is the segmentation mask for class i based on a probability map h.

2.3   Multi-phase Training Procedure

During the training process, the model was trained in three coarse-to-fine phases. For example, in the first phase of training, weights in unit 3 were updated, while weights in unit 2 and 1 were frozen; then in the second phase of training, weights in unit 2 were updated, while those in unit 3 and 1 were frozen. This multi-phase training procedure was employed to reduce the risk of overfitting for the whole model and it was based on our intuition that the output of each unit should function as a coarse estimation at its resolution. This regularization is helpful in our case for two reasons: (1) Our image data pool is limited even with random sampling and rotation-based data augmentation. (2) The ground truth is not necessarily reliable as manual segmentation in noisy 3D images is prone to errors. Similar methodology has been reported in several recent works [10].

2.4   Data Postprocessing

During the prediction step, the predicted probability map for the whole image was assembled together by summing all predicted patches with overlap while each patch is weighted by a Gaussian mask as specified in Eq. 1, since the model was trained to emphasize the performance at the center of the patch. Simple post processing was used to get rid of small anomalies in the predicted masks by setting the label of those anomalies whose volume were under a certain threshold to parenchyma.

3   Experiments and Results

3.1   Experiment Setup

The image data we used included 20 sets of multi-parameter 3D MR images, each of which consisted of one T2 weighted MR image and three T1 weighted dynamic enhanced contrast images at three different time points during the surgical intervention: pre-contrast phase (before the contrast injection), arterial

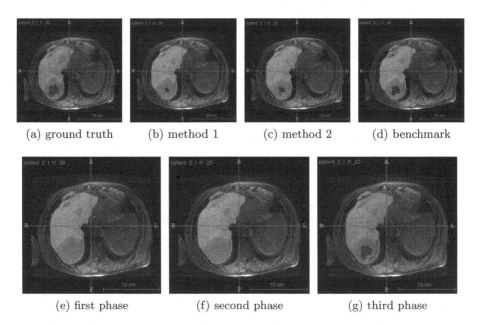

(a) ground truth   (b) method 1   (c) method 2   (d) benchmark

(e) first phase   (f) second phase   (g) third phase

Fig. 2. Segmentation demonstration. Red color is the parenchyma, green color is the viable tumor tissue, blue color is the necrosis. Subfigure 2a shows an expert delineation of some viable tumor tissue and necrosis. Subfigures 2b to d show the prediction results from three other methods, namely single-resolution input single-phase training, multi-resolution input single-phase training, and the benchmark method, manually designed features with random forest in auto-context, as described in Sect. 3.1. Subfigures 2e to g show the three-phase coarse-to-fine prediction progression in the proposed method. Visualization is provided using the software itk-SNAP. (Color figure online)

phase (20 s after the injection), and venous phase (70 s after the injection). All four images were mutually registered. Though a full automation that included liver segmentation was possible under our framework, liver masks were provided in order to achieve a fair comparison with the benchmark method, and to focus on the problem of the delineation inside the liver. Each patient's image intensity was normalized to roughly between 0 and 1.

Images used in this study are from HCC patients with TACE procedures as part of a larger clinical study on treatment outcome analysis. In these cases, the number of anomalies often ranges from 1 to 3, with diameter over 20 mm. During the TACE procedure, the largest tumors are the most important targets. Therefore the resolutions were selected as 2 mm, 1 mm and 1 mm, with a patch size of 16-by-16-by-16 voxels, in order to focus on performance on medium and large size tumors. The 20-patient dataset generated effectively 1700 non-overlapping patches, though with random sampling and random rotation augmentation, no patches would be exactly the same.

The first two units of the model were designed to differentiate anomalies from normal liver tissue, while the last one was designed to identify viable tumor tissue inside each detected anomaly. This was done by tuning the class weight ω in the loss function (Eq. 1). In phase 1, the ω's for parenchyma, viable tumor tissue, and necrosis are (1.0, 2.0, 0.3), phase 2 (1.0, 1.5, 0.3), and phase 3 (0.0, 1.0, 2.0). For each unit in the model, we implemented a U-net CNN with ten layers of $3 \times 3 \times 3$ convolution, ten layers of dropout, and two levels of max-pooling/upsampling. Five fold cross validation method was used to evaluate the performance of different models. Hyperparameters, such as learning rate and class weights in the loss functions, remained the same across all five folds.

3.2   A Combination of Measurements

In our evaluation of the method, we also included a two-step measurement instead of solely the traditional dice similarity coefficient (DSC). First, we calculated how well the anomalies were detected using F score (Eq. 3).

$$F_\beta = \frac{(1+\beta^2) \cdot true\ positive}{(1+\beta^2) \cdot true\ positive + \beta^2 \cdot false\ positive + false\ negative} \quad (3)$$

We set $\beta = 2$ to reflect the emphasis on recall rate in a clinical setting. An anomaly is detected if part of its voxels are covered by some predicted masks. Second, we measured how good the delineation was by aggregating all regions of interest (anomalies and viable tumor tissue) together and calculating the DSC. We provide a toy example to further explain the difference between the detection metric and the delineation metric in Fig. 3.

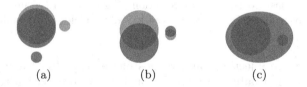

(a)   (b)   (c)

Fig. 3. Examples of difference between detection and delineation. Blue regions stand for anomalies. Orange regions stand for predictions. Subfigure (a): good delineation (high DSC), poor detection (low F score). Subfigure (b): medium delineation, good detection. Subfigure (c): poor delineation, good detection. (Color figure online)

3.3   Results

Figure 2 demonstrates an example of the proposed algorithm output. Table 1 summarizes the results in our study. The different rows in the method column describe whether the model utilized multi-resolution input, or only the resolution at the lowest level; whether it trained the model with a multi-phase strategy, or without. The single-resolution input single-phase training method is equivalent to the traditional U-net method. The benchmark method uses manually designed image features with random forest and iteratively trained auto-context classifiers

Table 1. Evaluation of different methods using a set of measurements.

method	Delineation: DSC		detection: F score
	Anomaly mass	Viable tumor tissue	
Multi-resolution input Multi-phase training	0.77	0.63	0.80
Multi-resolution input single-phase training	0.66	0.43	0.83
Single-resolution input single-phase training	0.68	0.48	0.81
Benchmark method	0.72	0.62	0.79

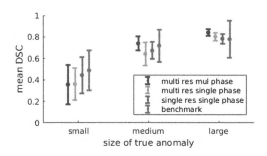

Fig. 4. Models' ability to delineate anomalies vs. their sizes. Small anomalies: $< 25\,\mathrm{mm}$ diameter, medium: $25 - 40\,\mathrm{mm}$, large: $> 40\,\mathrm{mm}$.

as described in [7]. Figure 4 describes how well the different models delineate anomalies at different sizes.

We make several observations from the results we present here.

1. The proposed method achieved the best overall anomaly and viable tumor tissue delineation performance, compared to both other CNN-based methods and the benchmark method.
2. The proposed method was tuned towards and did achieve the best performance in delineating medium and large size anomalies which the TACE procedure was targeting.
3. The proposed method was highly efficient in implementation. The whole model was trained within 90 min without the need of manually designing complex image features, while it took 18 hours for the benchmark method to finish running on a better machine.

4   Conclusion

In this work we presented a deep neural network approach to detect and delineate different types of liver tissue on multi-parameter MR images in patients with HCC. The patch-based algorithm was able to achieve a performance level that was better than the benchmark method without the need of manually designing different shape and texture features, with an implementation that was much more efficient. The multi-resolution input, the auto-context design and the multi-phase training procedure were helpful in improving overall performance compared to the traditional U-net architecture. In the future, this method can be applied to a full delineation of the liver tissue with any number of hierarchical tissue types, including the liver itself. In addition, this methodology can be applied to a number of other detection and delineation problems in the biomedical imaging field.

References

1. Christ, P.F., et al.: Automatic liver and lesion segmentation in CT using cascaded fully convolutional neural networks and 3D conditional random fields. In: Ourselin, S., Joskowicz, L., Sabuncu, M.R., Unal, G., Wells, W. (eds.) MICCAI 2016. LNCS, vol. 9901, pp. 415–423. Springer, Cham (2016). https://doi.org/10.1007/978-3-319-46723-8_48
2. Li, W., Jia, F., Hu, Q.: Automatic segmentation of liver tumor in CT images with deep convolutional neural networks. J. Comput. Commun. **3**(11), 146 (2015)
3. Raoul, J.L., et al.: Evolving strategies for the management of intermediate-stage hepatocellular carcinoma: available evidence and expert opinion on the use of transarterial chemoembolization. Cancer Treat. Rev. **37**(3), 212–220 (2011)
4. Raza, A., Sood, G.K.: Hepatocellular carcinoma review: current treatment, and evidence-based medicine. World J. Gastroenterol. WJG **20**(15), 4115 (2014)
5. Ronneberger, O., Fischer, P., Brox, T.: U-net: convolutional networks for biomedical image segmentation. In: Navab, N., Hornegger, J., Wells, W.M., Frangi, A.F. (eds.) MICCAI 2015. LNCS, vol. 9351, pp. 234–241. Springer, Cham (2015). https://doi.org/10.1007/978-3-319-24574-4_28
6. Salehi, S.S.M., Erdogmus, D., Gholipour, A.: Auto-context convolutional neural network (auto-net) for brain extraction in magnetic resonance imaging. IEEE Trans. Med. Imaging **36**(11), 2319–2330 (2017)
7. Treilhard, J., et al.: Liver tissue classification in patients with hepatocellular carcinoma by fusing structured and rotationally invariant context representation. In: Descoteaux, M., Maier-Hein, L., Franz, A., Jannin, P., Collins, D.L., Duchesne, S. (eds.) MICCAI 2017. LNCS, vol. 10435, pp. 81–88. Springer, Cham (2017). https://doi.org/10.1007/978-3-319-66179-7_10
8. Tu, Z., Bai, X.: Auto-context and its application to high-level vision tasks and 3D brain image segmentation. IEEE Trans. Pattern Anal. Mach. Intell. **32**(10), 1744–1757 (2010)
9. Vodopivec, T., Lepetit, V., Peer, P.: Fine hand segmentation using convolutional neural networks. CoRR abs/1608.07454 (2016). http://arxiv.org/abs/1608.07454
10. Zeng, G., Yang, X., Li, J., Yu, L., Heng, P.-A., Zheng, G.: 3D U-net with multi-level deep supervision: fully automatic segmentation of proximal femur in 3D MR images. In: Wang, Q., Shi, Y., Suk, H.-I., Suzuki, K. (eds.) MLMI 2017. LNCS, vol. 10541, pp. 274–282. Springer, Cham (2017). https://doi.org/10.1007/978-3-319-67389-9_32

Using 1D Patch-Based Signatures for Efficient Cascaded Classification of Lung Nodules

Dario Augusto Borges Oliveira$^{(\boxtimes)}$ and Matheus Palhares Viana

IBM Research Brazil, Rua Tutóia, 1157, Paraíso, São Paulo, Brazil
dariobo@br.ibm.com

Abstract. In the last years, convolutional neural networks (CNN) have been largely used to address a wide range of image analysis problems. In medical imaging, their importance increased exponentially despite of known difficulties in building large annotated training datasets in medicine. When it comes to 3D image exams analysis, 3D convolutional networks commonly represent the state-of-art, but can easily became computationally prohibitive due to the massive amount of data and processing involved. This scenario creates opportunities for methods that deliver competitive results while promoting efficiency in data usage and processing time. In this context, this paper proposes a comprehensive 1D patch-based data representation model to be used in an efficient cascaded approach for lung nodules false positive reduction. The proposed pipeline combines three convolutional networks: a 3D network that uses regular multi-scale volumetric patches, a 2D network that uses a trigonometric bi-dimensional representation of these patches, and a 1D network that uses a very compact 1D patch representation for filtering obvious cases. We run our experiments using the publicly available LUNA challenge dataset and demonstrate that the proposed cascaded approach achieves very competitive results while using up to **55 times less data** in average and running around **3.5 times faster** in average when compared to regular 3D CNNs.

Keywords: Convolutional neural networks · Deep learning
Dimension reduction · Medical imaging · Lung nodules

1 Introduction

Convolutional neural networks (CNNs) are widely used for image analysis in many different fields for a variety of purposes. In medical imaging they support image segmentation and classification, exams retrieval, and aid in diagnosis in general, aiming at assisting specialists to analyze more exams in less time with higher precision. Extensive reviews of deep learning usage in medical imaging can be found in the literature [4, 7].

© Springer Nature Switzerland AG 2018
W. Bai et al. (Eds.): Patch-MI 2018, LNCS 11075, pp. 67–75, 2018.
https://doi.org/10.1007/978-3-030-00500-9_8

Considering 2D image analysis, CNNs leveraged performance in classification and segmentation to very high standards, and close to real-time testing performances. When it comes to 3D high-definition exams, however, many usual architectures struggle with the associated computational cost and data usage. This scenario creates opportunities for innovative CNN-based methods that reduce the computational cost of 3D image analysis but still deliver competitive accuracy performance when compared to full 3D models.

In this context, this paper presents an innovative cascaded multi-scale approach that combines three different networks using different data representations: a regular 3D CNN that uses three different scales of volumetric patches around a point candidate; a 2D CNN proposed by [5] that uses a comprehensive bi-dimensional patch representation that achieves better performance in comparison to regular orthonormal planes; and a 1D CNN herein proposed that subsamples the bi-dimensional patches into a 1D very compact signature, that is used to filter more obvious candidates. In this approach all candidates are evaluated by the 1D network, tricky candidates are passed to the 2D network that further evaluate them, and hard cases are evaluated by the 3D network. This way we create a pipeline that delivers a fast and low data usage alternative targeting at real-time micro-services for patch-based nodule analysis.

We tested our approach using the lung nodule false positive (FP) reduction track in the publicly available data of LUNA (LUng Nodule Analysis) challenge and achieved over benchmark results using less data and running faster in comparison to regular 3D CNNs. Our results show the potential of our method, and results from an extensive list of methods using the same data and experiment design can be found in [6].

The remainder of this paper is organized as follows: in Sect. 2 we briefly describe our cascaded approach and the data representation used in each CNN. Then, we describe our experiments in Sect. 3 and present our results and discussions in Sect. 4. Finally, conclusions are drawn in Sect. 5.

2   Methodology

Traditionally, tools for aid in lung nodules detection use image processing techniques to generate a large number of candidates to be further analyzed [6]. Formally, a given q-th nodule candidate might be represented by its position in 3D, $\mathbf{r}_q = (i_q, j_q, k_q)$ and its label $\ell_q \in [0, 1]$, where $\ell_q = 0$ indicates a false nodule and $\ell_q = 1$ indicates a true nodule. Classification methods filter the list of candidates and narrow it down to strong candidates that should be visually inspected by a specialist. An usual bottleneck in the process happens when the number of candidates remaining to be checked (false positives) is too high. In this context, LUNA challenge proposed a track to reduce this bottleneck and foster the development of methods for lung nodule false positive reduction.

2.1   3D CNN Data Representation

An usual pipeline for FP reduction consists in going through a list of nodule candidates, sampling patches using their neighbouring volume, and classifying the patches. The most intuitive way of representing a volumetric patch of interest in medical imaging is to sample a cube of size $\sim \delta^3$ centered at a point of interest. This sampling is spatially coherent and contains all the raw data information within a defined neighborhood but is usually very inefficient both in terms of memory usage and the computational cost when using 3D CNNs.

2.2   2D CNN Data Representation

To overcome computational performance issues, many approaches (as reported in [6]) propose to sample the 3D neighbourhood of a given voxel by means of 2D cross sections of size $\sim \delta^2$ corresponding to its axial, coronal and sagittal views. Such representation provides an overview of the voxel neighbourhood and requires lower computational cost and memory usage compared to the 3D sampling. However, this sampling approach leaves much of the 3D information behind and usually delivers poor results in comparison to 3D models. Some alternatives like [2], propose using several planes randomly oriented to get more information, at the cost of increasing data usage and computational burden.

In [5], a data representation method was proposed to sample volumetric patches by means of comprehensive curved bi-dimensional patches, proven to allow better performance in 2D CNNs classification. In this paper, we extend this representation and deliver a very compact 1D signature to represent 3D patches.

The basal data representation method proposed by [5] uses a parametric function shown in Eq. 1 to visit the N sampling points $\mathbf{u} = (x, y, z)$ in the neighbourhood of a candidate $\mathbf{r} = (i, j, k)$. In Eq. 1, $t \in [0, N - 1]$, and the sampling rate is determined by N and the frequency ω. Figure 1-I-B illustrates the sampling points for $N = 150$ and $\omega = 50$, generating 3 blades.

$$\begin{bmatrix} z \\ x \\ y \end{bmatrix} = \begin{bmatrix} 2t/(N-1) - 1 \\ \sin\left(\arccos\left(z\right)\right)\cos\left(z\omega\pi\right) \\ \sin\left(\arccos\left(z\right)\right)\sin\left(z\omega\pi\right) \end{bmatrix} \tag{1}$$

For each sampling point $\mathbf{u} = (x, y, z)$, a line segment that goes from $\mathbf{r} - \frac{1}{2}\delta\mathbf{u}$ to $\mathbf{r} + \frac{1}{2}\delta\mathbf{u}$ is computed. The parameter δ defines the length of the line segments and ultimately the size of the neighborhood of $\mathbf{u}$ to be sampled. Finally, intensities are probed from the 3D volume along the line segments as shown in Fig. 1-I-B/C. The sampling points and the corresponding line segments form $b = N/\omega$ blades in the xy-axis projection. Figure 1-C shows one of the three blades obtained for the configuration $N = 150$ and $\omega = 50$.

Line segments belonging to the same blade are stacked side-by-side to generate b 2D patches of size $\omega \times \delta$. In our cascaded method experiments, we used $N = 150$ and $\omega = 50$, resulting in $b = 3$ blades. Examples of cross section views

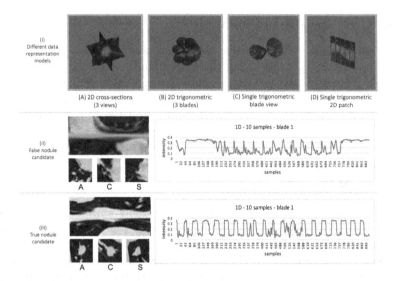

Fig. 1. Data representation using our method considering 3-blades and the usual axial, coronal and sagittal cross-sections at three different scales.

and corresponding trigonometric patches are shown in Fig. 1-II/III-left. Considering a roughly spherical high-intensity nodule, Fig. 1-III-left depicts a bright circular area in the usual cross-section views, and a bright central area in the transformed 2D trigonometric patch. A given false nodule candidate shown in Fig. 1-II-left, appears as an irregular object in both the trigonometric patch and its corresponding cross-section views.

2.3   1D CNN Data Representation

To extend the trigonometric 2D data representation we derived a simple yet highly compressed 1D signature from the 2D trigonometric patches: we use a regular grid over the bi-dimensional image and visit it column-wise, concatenating the samples in a single vector. This is equivalent to sample rays crossing the nodule candidate center, ordered by an uniform tri-dimensional trigonometric curve. More specifically, each 1D signature corresponds to the intensity along evenly spaced line segments defined by a given trigonometric patch, as highlighted by the red lines in Fig. 1-I-C/D.

One can notice that 1D signatures of true nodules and false nodules are very different (and therefore highly discriminant), as illustrated by the signatures examples shown in Fig. 1-II/III-right. The true nodule signature resembles as rough square wave, while false nodules present more complex patterns.

2.4   CNN Architecture

Through all our experiments we used the Xception architecture proposed by [1] for binary classification. We also created an equivalent 3D model by replacing the 2D convolutional layers by 3D convolutional layers, and an equivalent 1D model by replacing the 2D convolutional layers by 1D convolutional layers. We used these three architectures to compare the performance between our cascaded approach, the usual 3D CNN, the cross-section 2D CNN, the trigonometric 2D CNN, and the 1D signature CNN in the context of the LUNA false positive reduction track.

2.5   Our Cascaded Approach

To fully benefit from such compact data representation, we propose a cascaded schema, where we evaluate samples by demand and deliver a highly accurate yet efficient classification pipeline, shown in Fig. 2. In this approach, we begin evaluating all nodule candidates using their 1D signatures using the very efficient 1D network. Then, we check the outcome and remove all nodules with likelihood of being a nodule less than a threshold E (in our experiments we tested E equal to 1%, 5% and 10%), considered to be correctly classified as non-nodules. We generate the bi-dimensional trigonometric patches from the remaining nodule candidates and feed them to a 2D CNN, and then check the outcome and filter nodules with likelihood less than the pre-defined threshold. Finally, we submit the remaining nodules to the 3D network and compile the final outcome.

This schema allow us to evaluate candidates with high probability of being a nodule using very accurate 3D networks, while filtering many of the obvious non-nodule candidates using much more efficient networks. Figure 2 illustrate the process, and show the gains in data usage and processing time in each step. We show further benefits of such approach in the results section.

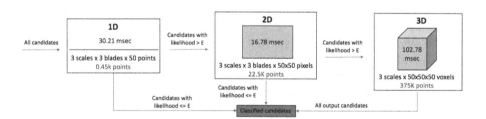

Fig. 2. Our cascaded approach: nodule candidates are fed to a 1D network, obvious non-nodules are filtered, remaining nodules are further evaluated by a 2D network. Again, obvious non-nodule candidates are filtered, and the remaining ones are evaluated by the very accurate 3D network. Such schema delivers highly accurate and efficient results.

3   Experiments Design

3.1   Data

The data used in our experiments was made publicly available by the LUNA 2016 challenge [6]. The LIDC/IDRI database is composed by 888 CT scans with nodule annotations provided by different specialists for nodules with diameter greater than 3 mm.

As pre-processing, we extracted 3D patches from the CT exams in three different scales: 10 mm × 10 mm × 10 mm, 25 mm × 25 mm × 25 mm and 40 mm × 40 mm × 40 mm, each of them sampled as 50 × 50 × 50 patches. Each scale was represented as a different channel, meaning that final 3D patches have 50 × 50 × 50 × 3 = 375 k voxels. We also created 2D data representations from these 3D patches using the trigonometric sampling approach used in this paper, and regular cross-sections for comparison matters, generating 150 × 50 × 3 = 22.5 k pixels images, where 3 is the number of cross-sections/blades used, and 150 are the three scales concatenated. For 1D signatures, we sub-sampled the trigonometric patches and generated a single 450 positions array, composed by 50 samples per patch, per scale, all concatenated with a 5 pixels spacing regular grid.

3.2   Training and Testing Procedures

The CNN models were trained using the 10-fold cross-validation schema proposed in LUNA challenge. For each fold we used nine subsets for training, and the remaining one for testing the trained model. In our experiments, we used 1 subset of the training data for validation and Adam for weights optimization. We trained our models in two sequences of 20 epochs, and augmented the nodule class samples using the random rotations. We also sub-sampled at random the non-nodule class to balance the training dataset, comprising a total of 75000 samples per epoch evenly balanced. During the test we provided 3 different samples for each nodule candidate by rotating at random the sample for each model, averaging the outcome. This way we avoid penalizing candidates with a controversial orientation.

The LUNA challenge evaluation tool was used for the final score. In this tool, each cross-validation fold was submitted to the corresponding trained model and compiled into a single 10-folds table that was evaluated using the script provided by the challenge. The script implements the free receiver operation characteristic (FROC) analysis and uses a bootstrap with 95% confidence interval to set different thresholds on the raw prediction probabilities, to deliver the percentage of average number of false positives per scan. Details are provided in [6].

4   Results and Discussion

Our experiments aimed at evaluating the benefits of using the proposed 1D signatures in a cascaded approach and to compare with other usual models. We evaluated the models accuracy in terms of false positive reduction rate and also analyzed the performance in terms of data usage and execution time. Note that the analysis of other CNN architectures and an extensive analysis of Xception architecture parameters could potentially improve results, but this is beyond the scope of this paper.

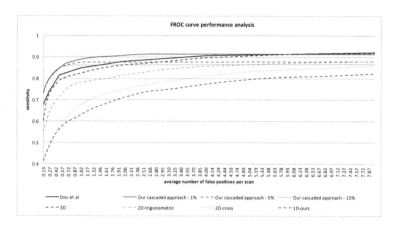

Fig. 3. FROC curves representing the performance of our method compared to 3D patches, trigonometric patches, cross-sections patches, the proposed one-dimensional signatures and the available state-of-art in the literature.

Our results show that the cascaded schema herein proposed delivers superior performance when compared to 3D CNNs, CNNs using 2D trigonometric patches proposed by [5], CNNs using regular 2D cross-section patches and CNNs using only the 1D signatures also presented in this paper. It also performed better than the current benchmark ([3]) for lung nodules false positive reduction, which demonstrates the potential of such approach. These results are compiled in Fig. 3.

In terms of processing time, our approach evaluated candidates **3.5 faster** than a regular 3D CNN, while using up to **50 times less data**. We also noticed that increasing the threshold E saves a great amount of data usage, but represents a drop in accuracy, as expected and shown by the red curves in Fig. 3.

Table 1. Accuracy at 2 false positives per exam, data usage, and execution time per testing sample (including sampling time) in different configurations using a K40 GPU.

Method	Acc@2FP	Data usage	Proc. time per sample
Dou et al. [3]	0.878	–	–
3D CNN	0.862	375 k	102.87 ms
2D-trigonometric CNN [5]	0.814	22.5 k	**16.78 ms**
2D-cross-sections CNN	0.749	22.5 k	16.85 ms
1D-proposed CNN	0.709	0.45 k	30.21 ms
Our cascaded approach 1%	**0.907**	17.86 k	29.99 ms
Our cascaded approach 5%	0.876	8.93 k	30.08 ms
Our cascaded approach 10%	0.863	**6.9 k**	30.19 ms

An interesting counter intuitive phenomenon was observed when we noticed that 1D CNNs processing time is higher than the ones observed in 2D CNNs. We believe this is related to two aspects: first, sampling 1D signatures is slower: we sample the trigonometric patch, than we extract the signatures; second, the 2D Xception architecture is optimized to run 1D convolutions, so processing time results were expected to be highly competitive. Even if we decided to prioritize data usage targeting micro-services, and evaluated the 1D signatures first in the cascaded schema, one could easily alter its order and run the 2D analysis first to prioritize processing time saving (Table 1).

5   Conclusions

This paper presents a very compact patch-based data representation model to be used within a cascaded approach for lung nodules false positive reduction. We extend the trigonometric patch data representation method presented in [5], and propose a method for generating one-dimensional signatures that derive highly accurate results while saving data usage and processing time.

We run several experiments to demonstrate the suitability of our approach for efficient CNN-based volumetric patch classification. We managed to deliver over benchmark results (0.907 acc@2FP in our best configuration against 0.878 with most commonly documented benchmark method) using up to **55 times less data** in average and running around **3.5 times faster** in average when compared to a single 3D CNN. These results seem to support our initial hypothesis that compact data representation can be used for filtering obvious cases and improve overall performance and efficiency if used on-demand with state-of-art approaches.

Further work would probably involve exploring different functions for modelling the data representation and improving the CNN architecture itself to increase performance using compact data representations.

References

1. Chollet, F.: Xception: Deep learning with depthwise separable convolutions. In: IEEE Conference on Computer Vision and Pattern Recognition, pp. 1251–1258 (2017)
2. Ciompi, F., et al.: Towards automatic pulmonary nodule management in lung cancer screening with deep learning. arXiv preprint arXiv:1610.09157 (2016)
3. Dou, Q., Chen, H., Yu, L., Qin, J., Heng, P.A.: Multi-level contextual 3D CNNs for false positive reduction in pulmonary nodule detection. IEEE Trans. Biomed. Eng. **PP**(99), 1 (2016)
4. Litjens, G., et al.: A survey on deep learning in medical image analysis. Med. Image Anal. **42**(Supplement C), 60–88 (2017). http://www.sciencedirect.com/science/article/pii/S1361841517301135
5. Oliveira, D.A.B., Viana, M.P.: An efficient multi-scale data representation method for lung nodule false postive reduction using convolutional neural networks. In: IEEE International Symposium on Biomedical Imaging (ISBI 2018). IEEE (2018)

6. Setio, A.A.A., et al.: Validation, comparison, and combination of algorithms for automatic detection of pulmonary nodules in computed tomography images: the LUNA16 challenge. Med. Image Anal. **42**, 1–13 (2017). https://doi.org/10.1016/j.media.2017.06.015
7. Tajbakhsh, N., et al.: convolutional neural networks for medical image analysis: full training or fine tuning? IEEE Trans. Med. Imaging **35**(5), 1299–1312 (2016)

Predicting Future Bone Infiltration Patterns in Multiple Myeloma

Roxane Licandro[1,2(✉)], Johannes Hofmanninger[2], Marc-André Weber[3],
Bjoern Menze[4], and Georg Langs[2]

[1] Institute of Visual Computing and Human-Centered Technology - Computer Vision
Lab, TU Wien, Vienna, Austria
roxane.licandro@meduniwien.ac.at
[2] Department of Biomedical Imaging and Image-guided Therapy - Computational
Imaging Research Lab, Medical University of Vienna, Vienna, Austria
[3] Institute of Diagnostic and Interventional Radiology, University Medical Center
Rostock, Rostock, Germany
[4] Institute of Biomedical Engineering - Image-Based Biomedical Modelling,
Technische Universität München, Munich, Germany

Abstract. Multiple Myeloma (MM) is a bone marrow malignancy
affecting the generation pathway of plasma cells and B-lymphocytes. It
results in their uncontrolled proliferation and malignant transformation
and ultimately can lead to osteolytic lesions first visible in MRI. The ear-
liest possible reliable detection of these lesions is critical, since they are
a prime marker of disease advance and a trigger for treatment. However,
their detection is difficult. Here, we present and evaluate a methodology
to predict future lesion emergence based on T1 weighted Magnetic Resonance Imaging (MRI) patch data. We train a predictor to identify early
signatures of emerging lesions before they reach thresholds for reporting.
The algorithm proposed uses longitudinal training data, and visualises
high- risk locations in the bone structure.

1 Introduction

Multiple Myeloma (MM) accounts for 10% of all bone marrow malignancies with
an incidence rate of 6/100000 per year in western countries [5]. It is the second
most common blood affecting malignancy, which disturbs the generation pathway of plasma cells and B-lymphocytes. Consequently, these cells proliferate
uncontrolled and are transformed in a malignant way [10]. In addition, the pro-
duction of large amounts of non-functional monoclonal antibodies is enforced,
which affects the function of kidneys, increases the deficiency in immune response
and in an advanced stage, influences the generation of bone forming and resorb-
ing cells. MM starts at a precursor state of *Monoclonal Gammopathy of Under-
tmined Significance* (MGUS) and further envolves to an asymptomatic form of
the disease *smoldering Multiple Myeloma* (sMM) with a predictable progression
to the symptomatic form of MM [4].

© Springer Nature Switzerland AG 2018
W. Bai et al. (Eds.): Patch-MI 2018, LNCS 11075, pp. 76–84, 2018.
https://doi.org/10.1007/978-3-030-00500-9_9

Longitudinal bone infiltration patterns of MM progression. The increased amount of plasma cells in MM leads to the alteration of bone remodelling mechanisms, by promoting bone resorption and inhibiting bone formation [10]. This results first in the formation of focal or diffuse bone marrow infiltration. The gold standard for observing these initial infiltration patterns is MRI (T1, T2) [1,4,8]. Subsequently, the progression of the disease leads to the building of osseous destructions, which are observable using low-dose Computer Tomography (CT) [6]. Figure 1 illustrates the infiltration pattern of a focal lesion evolving at the distal part of the femur over three examination time points of a single patient.

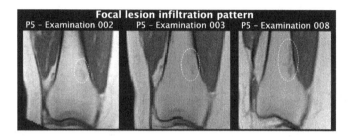

Fig. 1. Visualisation of an infiltration pattern of a focal lesion (yellow) using T1 weighted MRI scans over multiple examination time points of one patient.

Challenges. Challenges of tracking lesions over time are, identifying early signatures of their emergence, accurate alignment of subject whole body images, imaging artefacts, and subtle non rigid deformations, as well as capturing the heterogeneity of diffuse infiltration patterns and their imaging signatures. Different treatment strategies and patient specific treatment response, and progression speed cause further variability. According to the results reported in the recent study of Mateos et al. [7], it is particularly important to assess high-risk sMM patients for developing MM and corresponding infiltration patterns, since a benefit for the patient from early therapy is observable.

Contribution. Here, we propose and evaluate a predictor for future bone infiltration patterns. The algorithm uses longitudinal data to learn a local predictor of lesion emergence and change. We assess longitudinal relationships between subsequent stages of bone lesions and corresponding infiltration patterns of MM patients to provide a predictive signature for bone lesions. The contribution of the paper is three fold: (1) the longitudinal alignment of multiple bodyparts in whole body MRIs, (2) a classifier incorporating data from different disease stages in MM and (3) a local lesion risk score (LRS) to identify bone regions with a higher probability to evolve to diffuse or osteolytic lesions. We first give an overview of methodology and the data in Sect. 2. The evaluation results are presented in Sect. 3 and the conclusion of this work and possibilities for future work are summarized in Sect. 4.

2   Methodology

We first describe longitudinal alignment, and then introduce the methodology to estimate a local Lesion Risk Score (LRS) for future lesion emergence. Figure 2 illustrates the computation pipeline of the lesion risk score. It consists of four components: data acquisition, data preprocessing, train and test data design and LRS computation. Details regarding the train and test data design are summarized in Sect. 3.

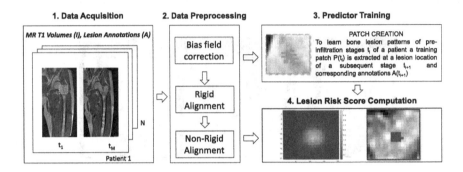

Fig. 2. Lesion Risk Score computation pipeline

Longitudinal Alignment. To perform subject specific longitudinal analysis of subsequent lesion states, we first register a patient's data $I_{t_i} = \{I_{t_1}, ... I_{t_M}\}$. A patient's image at a timepoint t_i is aligned to all subsequent timepoints $x = t_{i+1}, ..., t_M$, depending on the number of available data. Bias field correction is used to process imaging data before alignment using FAST[1] [3] integrated in the FMRIB Software Library (FSL)[2]. The aligned image $\overline{I_{t_i}(x)}$ is obtained following a two step registration procedure (cf. Eq. 1).

$$\overline{I_{t_i}(x)} = I_{t_i} \circ \phi_{NR}((A * I_{t_i}), I_x) \tag{1}$$

Although longitudinal data is registered, patients' shape vary over time, since the median inverval between MRIs is 13 months. Also the acquired images do not visualise exactly the same body part snippets. Thus, we decided (based on experimental results), to use an affine approach first. This affine alignment A is performed using a block matching method for global registration. The resulting transformed image $(A * I_{t_1})$ is used as moving image in the second alignment step. Subsequently, a non-rigid deformation ϕ_{NR} to the target at time point x is estimated. For affine registration the function *reg_aladin* and for non rigid alignment the function *reg_f3d* are used, which are integrated in the NiftyReg toolbox[3] [9]. For assessing the quality of registration, moving and target image

---

[1] https://fsl.fmrib.ox.ac.uk/fsl/fslwiki/FAST [accessed 11th of June 2018].

[2] https://fsl.fmrib.ox.ac.uk/fsl/fslwiki/FSL [accessed 11th of June 2018].

[3] http://cmictig.cs.ucl.ac.uk/research/software/software-nifty/niftyreg [accessed 11th of June 2018].

were inspected manually using overlay visualisations and evaluated regarding correspondence of lesions' position between the different time points.

Patch Creation and Data Augmentation. After alignment, MR images $\overline{I_{t_1}(x)}$ of a patient correspond to timepoints x and corresponding annotations S_x of the lesion in a future image of the patient. After the longitudinal alignment of acquisitions of one patient, datasets are created by using the intensity image of a subject at time point t and to this time point aligned annotations of lesions of subsequent time points $t + i$, where i is $1, ..., n$ (n... number of available subsequent time points). Given those data pairs, patches are created in the lesion regions, by first computing the barycentre of the lesion's annotation in the subsequent state and randomly moving a clipping window around it to avoid the predictor to learn uniform lesion positions. Additionally, we repeated this procedure for rotated intensity images and corresponding annotations. The rotations were performed in 20 degree steps.

Local Lesion Risk Score. The proposed local Lesion Risk Score (LRS) uses early signatures of emerging bone lesions to predict future lesions and mark corresponding high risk locations. We use the computed pairs of image patches and corresponding lesion annotations of a subsequent state to train a random forest classifier that predicts future lesion labels from the present image patch data. During application, a score is obtained for each voxel position V by the probability predicted by the trained random forest for a new input patch.

$$LRS_V = P_{RF}(\overline{I_{t_i}(x)}) \tag{2}$$

We used the Python framework *sklearn* with an integrated Random Forest predictor[4] with 10 decision trees and the following parametrisation: n_estimators = 10, criterion = 'gini', max_depth = 2, min_samples_split = 2, min_samples_leaf = 1, min_weight_fraction_leaf = 0.0, max_features = 'auto', max_leaf_nodes = None, min_impurity_decrease = 0.0, min_impurity_split = None, bootstrap = True, oob_score = False, n_jobs = 1, random_state = None, verbose = 0, warm_start = False, class_weight = None.

3   Results

In this section an overview of the evaluation dataset is given and the quantitative as well qualitative LRS evaluation results are presented and discussed.

Dataset. In this study 220 longitudinal whole body (wb) MRIs from 63 patients with smoldering multiple myeloma (following the 2003 guidelines [2]) were acquired between 2004 and 2011. At least one wbMRI was performed per patient. The annotation of focal lesions is performed manually by medical experts starting at a lesion size bigger than 5 mm [1], since according to the IMWG consensus statement, from this size on, patients are considered to have symptomatic

---

[4] http://scikit-learn.org/stable/modules/generated/sklearn.ensemble.
RandomForestClassifier.html [accessed 10th of June 2018].

myeloma with therapy requirement. Table 1 summarizes the study participant's demographics. The protocol of this study was approved by the institutional ethics committee and all subjects gave their informed consent prior to inclusion. The scanning was performed on a 1.5 Tesla Magnetom Avanto (Siemens Healthineers, Erlangen, Germany) scanner. For the T1 weighted acquisition a turbo spine echo sequence (repetition time (TR): 627 milliseconds (ms), echo time (TE): 11 ms, section thickness (ST): 5 mm, acquisition time (TA): 2:45 min) was performed of the head, thorax, abdomen, pelvis and legs using a coronal orientation and for the spine in sagital orientation. No contrast medium was given. The duration of a scan was approximately 40 min long.

Table 1. Participants' demographics

Patients	63 (24 female)
Therapy	Radiation or resection
Median age at initial MRI (yrs)	55
Age range (yrs)	29–76
Median interval between MRIs	13 months
Median observation time	46 months

Train and Test Data Design. In this study we used acquisitions from two body regions: In *region 1* thorax, abdomen and pelvis are visualised and in *region 2* the lower part of the pelvis, femurs and knees. These areas are considered since most lesions occur in those. In this work we observe two types of lesions and evaluate the performance of the methodology proposed separately for every type, with corresponding train and test sets: lesions which are *emerging*, i.e. which are not reported in the first scan, but in the subsequent scan, and *changing* lesions, which are annotated at both observed examination time points. For every patient we extracted image patches at lesion regions longitudinally over subsequent states of three different sizes ($10 \times 4 \times 10$, $20 \times 4 \times 20$ and $30 \times 4 \times 30$ voxels with a voxelspacing of $1.302\,mm \times 6\,mm \times 1.302\,mm$). To obtain a higher number of patches for the predictor training, data augmentation is performed resulting in *18 different patches per lesion*. To summarize, for emerging lesions we obtain 720 patches for region 1 and 504 patches for region 2 and for growing lesions we created 1026 patches for region 1 and 810 patches for region 2. Crossvalidation is used to generate test and training datasets, where a testset consists of 18 patches of a single lesion including the volumes of different orientation, which results in 40 folds for emerging lesions in region 1 and 28 in region 2 and 57 folds for growing lesion in region 1 and 45 in region 2.

Evaluation Setup. For the quantitative evaluation and for obtaining comparability between the different tested setups, the Area Under the Curve (AUC) is computed, based on the probability estimates of the local lesion risk predictor for the test patch using scikit learn[5]. We used thresholding to obtain a predicted label for visualisation and comparison. We have to point out that an exact matching of predicted label and subsequent annotation is not achievable, given a pre-stage and not required since we aim to predict risk of lesion growth or emergence and not to estimate exact segmentations of future lesions.

Table 2. Summary results LRS performance

Lesion Type	Patch Size	Mean AUC Region 1	Mean AUC Region 2
Emerging	$10 \times 4 \times 10$	0.7425	0.769
	$20 \times 4 \times 20$	0.7003	0.7144
	$30 \times 4 \times 30$	0.6739	0.6874
Changing	$10 \times 4 \times 10$	0.7607	0.7221
	$20 \times 4 \times 20$	0.7104	0.7491
	$30 \times 4 \times 30$	0.6976	0.7096

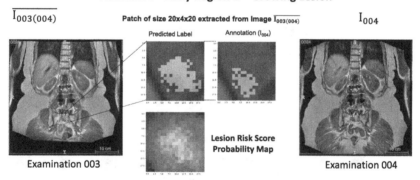

Patient 24 – Body Region 1 – Growing Lesion

$I_{003(004)}$ Patch of size 20x4x20 extracted from Image $I_{003(004)}$ I_{004}

Predicted Label   Annotation (I_{004})

Lesion Risk Score Probability Map

Examination 003   Examination 004

Fig. 3. Prediction of lesion growth from examination time point to time point in body region 1. The predicted label is visualised in the second column, below the underlying Local Lesion Risk Score probability map is shown and the manual annotation is visualised in the third column.

3.1 Evaluation Body Region 1

In Table 2 in column three the mean AUC for emerging and growing lesion types for body region 1 are summarized. For every lesion type three different patch sizes are evaluated. Figure 3 illustrates a prediction result for a growing lesion of a region 1 acquisition. The test image (left) is a transformed image from

---

[5] http://scikit-learn.org/stable/auto_examples/model_selection/plot_roc.html [accessed 10th of June 2018].

examination time point 003 to 004 using the longitudinal alignment approach introduced in Sect. 2. The extracted patch of this image in the region of the lesion visible in the image I_{003} is visualised in the first row in the center, with the predicted label in the second column and the annotation of the future lesion position extracted from image I_{004} in the third column. In the second row the predicted probability map of the local lesion risk score is visualised, where yellow shows regions of high probability and blue of low probability.

3.2   Evaluation Body Region 2

In Table 2 in column four the mean AUC for emerging and growing lesion types for body region 2 are summarized. For every lesion type three different patch sizes are evaluated. Figure 4 illustrates a prediction result for an emerging lesion of a region 2 acquisition. The test image (left) is a transformed image from examination time point 002 to 003. The extracted patch of this image in the region of the lesion visible in the target image I_{002} (right) is visualised, with the predicted label in the second column and the annotation of the future lesion position extracted from image I_{003} in the third column. In the second row the predicted probability map of the local lesion risk score is visualised, where yellow shows regions of high probability and blue of low probability.

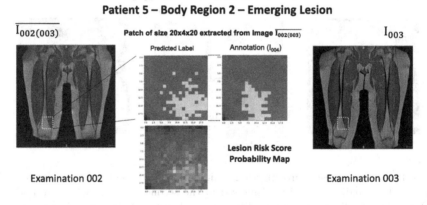

Fig. 4. Prediction of an emerging lesion from examination time point 002 to time point 003 in body region 2. The predicted label is visualised in column 2, below the underlying Local Lesion Risk Score probability map is shown and the manual annotation is visualised in column 3.

3.3   Discussion

For both lesion types a decrease of the mean AUC is observable with increasing patch size, where emerging lesions show a steeper decrease as growing lesions in both bodyparts. Also growing lesions in the femur, knees or pelvis are better predicted than those in the thoracic or abdominal body region.

4 Conclusion

In this work we present a local Lesion Risk Predictor for accessing and visualising regions of high risk for bone lesions to emerge or to grow. We trained a random forest predictor using lesion image patches and annotations of subsequent lesions states of the longitudinal MR T1 weighted dataset observed. The main challenge here was to achieve an accurate longitudinal alignment of subsequent examination time points of a patient. To our knowledge this is the first attempt to predict bone infiltration patterns in MM using T1 weighted MR images. Current approaches focus on lesion detection (e.g. [11] for CT images) using deep learning techniques. We decided to investigate a lesion predictor based on a random forest classifier first, since its setup, parametrisation and evaluation is simpler compared to deep learning approaches. However, we incorporated the possibility to extend the proposed patch based approach to evaluate deep architectures for lesion prediction in the future. To this point prediction using the introduced local lesion risk score is limited to image patches. For future work we aim to adapt the proposed score to be able to predict probability maps for entire volumes. Additionally, we will incorporate different modalities, and data from additional bodyparts in the framework proposed to longitudinally model infiltration and also osseous destruction patterns caused by the progress of multiple myeloma.

Acknowledgement. This work was supported by the Austrian Science Fund (FWF) project number I2714-B31

References

1. Dimopoulos, M.A., et al.: Role of magnetic resonance imaging in the management of patients with multiple myeloma: a consensus statement. J. Clin. Oncol. **33**(6), 657–664 (2015)
2. Durie, B.G.M., et al.: Myeloma management guidelines: a consensus report from the scientific advisors of the international Myeloma foundation. Hematol. J. **4**(6), 379–398 (2003)
3. Jenkinson, M., Beckmann, C.F., Behrens, T.E.J., Woolrich, M.W., Smith, S.M.: FSL. NeuroImage **62**(2), 782–90 (2012)
4. Kloth, J.K., et al.: Appearance of monoclonal plasma cell diseases in whole-body magnetic resonance imaging and correlation with parameters of disease activity. Int. J. Cancer **135**(10), 2380–2386 (2014)
5. Kyle, R.A., Rajkumar, S.V.: Multiple myeloma. Blood **111**(6), 2962–72 (2008)
6. Lambert, L., Ourednicek, P., Meckova, Z., Gavelli, G., Straub, J., Spicka, I.: Whole-body low-dose computed tomography in multiple myeloma staging: superior diagnostic performance in the detection of bone lesions, vertebral compression fractures, rib fractures and extraskeletal findings compared to radiography with similar radiation. Oncol. Lett. **13**(4), 2490–2494 (2017)
7. Mateos, M.-V., et al.: Lenalidomide plus dexamethasone versus observation in patients with high-risk smouldering multiple myeloma (QuiRedex): long-term follow-up of a randomised, controlled, phase 3 trial. Lancet. Oncol. **17**(8), 1127–1136 (2016)

8. Merz, M., et al.: Predictive value of longitudinal whole-body magnetic resonance imaging in patients with smoldering multiple myeloma. Leukemia **28**(9), 1902–1908 (2014)
9. Modat, M., Cash, D.M., Daga, P., Winston, G.P., Duncan, J.S., Ourselin, S.: Global image registration using a symmetric block-matching approach. J. Med. Imaging (Bellingham, Wash.) **1**(2), 024003 (2014)
10. Tosi, P.: Diagnosis and treatment of bone disease in multiple Myeloma: spotlight on spinal involvement. Scientifica, p. 104546
11. Xu, L., et al.: Automated whole-body bone lesion detection for multiple myeloma on 68 ga-pentixafor PET/CT imaging using deep learning methods. Contrast Media Mol. Imaging **2018**, 1–11 (2018)

A Fast Automatic Juxta-pleural Lung Nodule Detection Framework Using Convolutional Neural Networks and Vote Algorithm

Jiaxing Tan[1], Yumei Huo[1(✉)], Zhengrong Liang[2], and Lihong Li[1]

[1] City University of New York, New York City, NY, USA
jtan@gradcenter.cuny.edu, {Yumei.Huo,Lihong.Li}@csi.cuny.edu
[2] Stony Brook University, Stony Brook, NY, USA
Jerome.Liang@sunysb.edu

Abstract. Lung Nodule Detection from CT scans is a crucial task for the early detection of lung cancer with high difficulty performing an automatic detection. In this paper, we propose a fast automatic voting based framework using Convolutional Neural Network to detect juxta-pleural nodules, which are pulmonary (lung) nodules attached to the chest wall and hard to detect even by human experts. The detection result for each region in the CT scan is voted by the detection results of the extracted candidates from the region, which we formulate as a generative model. We perform two sets of experiments: one is to validate our framework, and the other is to compare different convolution neural network settings under our framework. The result shows our framework is competent to detect juxta-pleural lung nodules especially when only a weak classifier trained on noisy data is available. Meanwhile, we overcome the problem of determining the proper input size for nodules with high variance in diameters.

Keywords: Lung cancer · Juxta-pleural nodule detection
Deep learning· · Weakly labeled

1 Introduction

Lung cancer is the leading cause of cancer-related deaths in the United States [1]. Automated lung cancer detection is of great importance. In general, based on their locations, lung nodules can be classified into two types. One is juxta-pleural, which is typically attached to the lung wall; and the other one is the isolated type within the lung area. Compared with isolated nodules, juxta-pleural nodules are more difficult to detect because their intensities and texture are similar to those of the chest wall and they usually have relatively small radius. As a result, the traditional methods such as region growing [2] and active contour model [3],

© Springer Nature Switzerland AG 2018
W. Bai et al. (Eds.): Patch-MI 2018, LNCS 11075, pp. 85–92, 2018.
https://doi.org/10.1007/978-3-030-00500-9_10

usually fail in the classification of juxta-pleual nodules. Some examples of juxta-pleural nodules are shown in Fig. 1, where the red part is the labeled nodule by the radiologist.

Recently, Convolutional Neural Network (ConvNet) has achieved a great success in computer vision, especially in image classification with a fast updating accuracy score on the ImageNet Challenge since 2012 [4,5]. In contrast to the traditional feature-engineering, where machines use human hand-crafted features to learn, ConvNet is designed to have the machine learn features from data itself without human involvement. This makes the machine learning task more efficient as less pre-processing is needed. The success of ConvNet has cast some light on the area of bio-medical. Only in the area of bio-medical image scan analysis, ConvNet has already been applied to solve the problems such as organ segmentation [6,7], and lung nodule diagnosis [8]. Recently, Suzuki et al. [9] applied ConvNet for lung nodule detection and compared several different ConvNet designs.

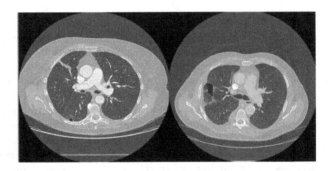

Fig. 1. Examples of juxta-pleural nodule from our dataset. The red color indicating the location and shape of nodules (Color figure online)

Traditionally, nodule detection pipeline requires a series of preprocessing, such as lung segmentation, vessel elimination, suspect candidates extraction and classification. On the other side, for a ConvNet based solution, it is tricky to find a proper input patch size to contain the whole nodules as it has high variance in diameter. Small nodules might be easily overlooked if the patch size is too small.

In this paper, we design a fast automatic voting based framework using Convolutional Neural Network to detect juxta-pleural nodules from raw CT scan. For each CT slice, we first divide the CT image into regions, where each region could be viewed as a bag of candidates. Then instead of throwing the whole region into ConvNet, we extract several candidates from each region and apply a voting algorithm to decide whether a nodule exists in that region or not. In addition, we compare our ConvNet with two ConvNet structures which have the highest AUC from [9] in terms of the performance on our juxta-pleural dataset. We perform two sets of experiments: one is to validate our framework and the other is to compare different ConvNet designs under our framework. Our experimental results show that the framework is efficient and our ConvNet structure outperforms the ones from [9] especially when only weakly labeled data with noise is available for training. Our voting algorithm could improve the original model by a large margin.

There are three major strengths of our propose framework. First, our model does not need any pre-processings on the raw data. Secondly, with the design of patch-based voting framework, we eliminate the problem of window size selection as well as enhance model performance. At last, our voting framework could significantly improve original ConvNet model's performance and could be generalized to different kinds of ConvNets.

2   Methodology

We designed a bag-of-voting-candidates (BOVC) model to perform nodule detection. For a CT scan R, we assume it contains H regions, denoted as $R = R_1, R_2, ..., R_H$, where each region has size $M \times N$ and independent and identically distributed (i.i.d). We view each region R_i as a bag of K voting candidates $R_i = C_{i,1}, C_{i,2}, ..., C_{i,K}$, where $C_{i,j} = < x_{i,j}, y_{i,j} >$ is the jth candidate of region i containing a data patch $x_{i,j}$ with its corresponding label $y_{i,j}$. We further assume that each candidate is independently generated by a hidden variable ϕ_i, indicating the class distribution of region i. The total probability of this generative model could be written as:

$$P(R; \phi) = \prod_{i=1}^{H} P(R_i|\phi_i)P(\phi_i) = \prod_{i=1}^{H}\prod_{j=1}^{K} P(C_{i,j}|\phi_i)P(\phi_i) \qquad (1)$$

The major workflow of our framework is shown in Fig. 2. There are two steps, the first step is to generate candidate given a certain region, the second step is to generate detection result with our ConvNet based patch voting algorithm. We will introduce both steps accordingly in the rest of this section.

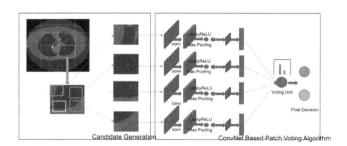

Fig. 2. Workflow of our framework, the first step is candidate extraction and the second step is our ConvNet based voting algorithm.

2.1   Candidate Extraction

We formulate our candidate generating algorithm as follow: For each region, take region i as an example, we extract k_1 candidates with size $T \times T$ ($T < min(M, N)$) from region i, where k_1 is set to make sure there are the least overlap to cover the whole region. Then we design to randomly extract k_2 more candidates to get more random votes. At last, we have K candidates in total. Then we perform translation on each candidate, which can further enrich dataset as well as provide more possible views of the candidate, as a result, several image patches (which will also be candidates) can be generated from a single original candidate.

2.2   Parameter Estimation with ConvNet

We design our parameter estimation algorithm with ConvNets. The two-step algorithm is described as follow:

Step1: We update the ConvNet parameter θ with regard to the following equation:

$$\theta = \arg\max_{\theta} P(R|\phi; \theta) = \arg\max_{\theta} P(R|\theta) = \arg\max_{\theta} \prod_{x_{i,j} \in R} P(x_{i,j}, y_i|\theta) \quad (2)$$

Step 2: Given θ, ϕ_i is estimated by:

$$\phi_{ij} = \frac{N_{ij}}{N_i}, \quad (3)$$

where N_{ij} is the count of candidates in region i predicted with label j by ConvNet and N_i is the total number of candidates in region i.

For our task, there are only two classes (nodule or non-nodule contained), denoted as positive and negative. Our vote algorithm generates the final decision for region i based on ϕ_i with the following rule:

$$Result(Region_i) = \begin{cases} Positive \ Ratio > Threshold \\ Negative \ Ratio < Threshold \end{cases} \quad (4)$$

The threshold in the equation is a predefined empirical value, which is the 15 percentile of the validation dataset and the ratio of region i is calculated as:

$$Ratio_i = \frac{\phi_{i,Possitive}}{\phi_{i,Possitive} + \phi_{i,Negative}} \quad (5)$$

ConvNet Design. The design of the ConvNet contains input layer, convolution layer, subsampling layer and fully connected layer. We design a ConvNet of input size 64×64 with two convolutional layers, each followed by a max-pooling layer. For the convolutional layer, we choose Leaky Rectified Linear Unit (LeakyReLU) [10] as the activation function:

$$LeakyReLU(x, \alpha) = max(x, 0) + \alpha \times min(x, 0),$$

where α is a small user pre-defined non-zero gradient negative slope that is set to negative values.

In Table 1, we detailed our ConvNet design with two ConvNet designs with the highest AUC in [9] as a comparison, which is denoted as sh-CNN and rd-CNN. The last column shows how many different kernels are used for a convolution layer or how many neurons are used in a fully connected layer. We are not specifying the input layer in the table since all ConvNets take input size of 64×64.

Table 1. Table of Different ConvNet Designs, here we compare three different designs, our proposed network, the one with the best performance from [9] and a very shallow model as comparisons.

Layer	Type	Kernel	No.	Layer	Type	Kernel	No.
(1) Our Model				(3) rd-CNN			
1	Convolution	7×7	32	1	Convolution	11×11	32
2	Max-pooling	2×2	-	2	Max-pooling	2×2	-
3	Convolution	5×5	64	3	Convolution	5×5	32
4	Max-pooling	2×2	-	4	Max-pooling	2×2	-
5	Fully connected	-	128	5	Convolution	3×3	32
6	Fully connected	-	2	6	Max-pooling	2×2	-
(2) sh-CNN				7	Convolution	3×3	64
1	Convolution	11×11	32	8	Max-pooling	2×2	-
2	Max-pooling	2×2	-	9	Fully connected	-	128
3	Fully connected	-	128	10	Fully connected	-	2
4	Fully connected	-	2				

A softmax fully-connected layer is used as the last layer to generate the probability distribution over two classes (Nodule and Non-Nodule). For the training of our ConvNet, cross-entropy Loss is used to minimize the difference between detected class and real class from groundtruth with L2 Norm regularization added. Note that in order to reuse training data, we design weight sharing among the separate ConvNet paths to make better use of the training data.

3 Experiments

The goal of the experiments is two-fold. One is to validate our framework, and the other is to compare different ConvNet designs under our framework.

3.1   Dataset

The original RAW CT data is acquired from the largest public database founded by the Lung Image Database Consortium and Image Database Resource Initiative (LIDC-IDRI). Each CT slice has a size of 512×512. Our radiologist labels the position of the nodule for each given CT slice.

We select 90 patients from our dataset with at least one juxta-pleural nodules included and has more than 12 slices containing nodules on average. By randomly sampling patches around nodule areas and non-nodule areas respectively, we obtain the positive samples and negative samples. And the rotation is applied as a translation method to each sample. In each patient's CT scan, the ratio of the nodule to non-nodule areas is now not balanced. However, to train a binary classifier, we have to use a balanced dataset, which means that there should be equal numbers of positive and negative samples. With regard to this point, we perform the last step to balance our training dataset.

3.2   Experiment Design

In our experiments, we choose the region size to be 128×128 and use rotation as the translation method. We extract $k = 9$ candidates from each region, which are patches located at 4 corners, 4 middle part on each edge, and 1 in the center. Apparently, there are some overlaps among the candidates. However, our candidate extraction method is more efficient than using a sliding window to cover the whole region. Each candidate will then be rotated 3 times.

We use Theano to implement ConvNet designs. For training, we apply Adam [11] optimizer with a batch size of 40. The learning rate is set to 10^{-4}, momentum to 0.9, and weight decay to 0.0005. The network is initialized with a Gaussian Distribution.

We designed two experiments to validate our framework. In the first experiment, we compare three models with and without voting algorithm to validate our framework on a test dataset containing 20 patients with a balanced number of positive and negative regions. The model without voting will consider each patch as a distinct input. And the voting result is achieved by our proposed model. We use AUC and F1 score as evaluation metrics for experiment 1. However, in practice, nodule detection is performed on highly unbalanced data. As a result, we designed second experiment to test our framework performance on 10 patients' CT slices containing nodules without balancing the dataset and use AUC for evaluation.

3.3   Experiment Result

The result of experiment 1 is shown in Fig. 3(a). It shows that vote algorithm has improved AUC for all ConvNet. And our model has a better performance than both rd-CNN and sh-CNN in both scenarios when the voting algorithm is used and not used respectively. Different from [9], sh-CNN has the worst performance on our dataset in both scenarios. Some typical highly confusing patches are shown in figure Fig. 4. We can see that most False Positive ones are caused by including the chest wall or some other tissues into the sampled patches, which increase the noise of data samples. On the other hand, the small size (radius) of a nodule is a major reason for True Negative ones.

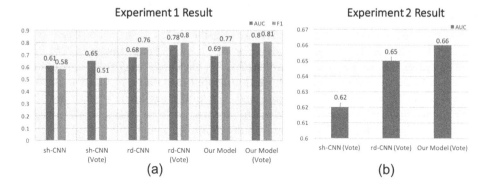

Fig. 3. Experiment result, (a) Performance comparison results in experiment 1 and (b) Performance comparison results in experiment 2.

In experiment 2, as the real detection has unbalanced data for two classes ($positive : neagtive > 1 : 20$), the performance is lower than that of experiment 1. The results are shown in Fig. 3(b). We can see that our model works the best, which is slightly better than rd-CNN, while sh-CNN has the lowest AUC.

In conclusion, our experiments showed that our automatic detection framework, which is based on ConvNet, can detect juxta-pleural lung nodule from CT scan of a patient efficiently. Especially when the effect of a detection classifier is limited by noisy training data, our vote algorithm could be used to enhance its performance.

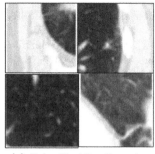

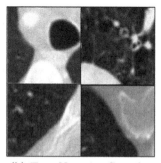

(a) False Positive Samples   (b) True Negative Samples

Fig. 4. Typical highly confusing samples in experiment 1

4   Conclusion and Future Work

In this paper, we propose a framework to detect juxta-pleural nodule from CT scans based on ConvNet using vote algorithm. We compared different ConvNet structures in our framework and examined the effectiveness of our framework on LIDC-IDRI juxta-pleural lung nodule datasets. Experiments show that our framework is competent at detecting juxta-pleural nodules. On the other side, our experiments show that the incorrectly classified data samples are those containing the chestwall or some noisy, so some preprocessing methods could be used to filter out those "bad" samples. A possible extension could be training different ConvNet with image patch randomly split into different groups. For our future work, besides the above mentioned continuing research, we will also try other ConvNet structures to enhance the accuracy of the classifier and design an efficient framework to locate the nodules from CT scans.

References

1. American Cancer Society: Key statistics for lung cancer (2016)
2. Adams, R., Bischof, L.: Seeded region growing. IEEE Trans. Pattern Anal. Mach. Intell. **16**(6), 641–647 (1994)
3. Kass, M., Witkin, A., Terzopoulos, D.: Snakes: active contour models. Int. J. Comput. Vis. **1**(4), 321–331 (1988)
4. Krizhevsky, A., Sutskever, I., Hinton, G.E.: Imagenet classification with deep convolutional neural networks. In: Advances in Neural Information Processing Systems, pp. 1097–1105 (2012)
5. Szegedy, C., et al.: Going deeper with convolutions. In: Proceedings of the IEEE Conference on Computer Vision and Pattern Recognition, pp. 1–9 (2015)
6. Li, R., Zeng, T., Peng, H., Ji, S.: Deep learning segmentation of optical microscopy images improves 3-D neuron reconstruction. IEEE Trans. Med. Imaging **36**(7), 1533–1541 (2017)
7. Cha, K.H., et al.: Urinary bladder segmentation in ct urography using deep-learning convolutional neural network and level sets. Med. Phys. **43**(4), 1882–1896 (2016)
8. Kumar, D., Wong, A., Clausi, D.A.: Lung nodule classification using deep features in ct images. In: 2015 12th Conference on Computer and Robot Vision (CRV), pp. 133–138. IEEE (2015)
9. Tajbakhsh, N., Suzuki, K.: Comparing two classes of end-to-end machine-learning models in lung nodule detection and classification: MTANNS vs. CNNS. Pattern Recognit. **63**, 476–486 (2017)
10. Maas, A.L., Hannun, A.Y., Ng, A.Y.: Rectifier nonlinearities improve neural network acoustic models
11. Kingma, D.P., Ba, J.: Adam: a method for stochastic optimization, arXiv preprint arXiv:1412.6980 (2014)

Brain Image Analysis

LesionBrain: An Online Tool for White Matter Lesion Segmentation

Pierrick Coupé[1,2(✉)], Thomas Tourdias[3,4,5], Pierre Linck[4,5],
José E. Romero[6], and José V. Manjón[6]

[1] CNRS, LaBRI, UMR 5800, PICTURA, 33400 Talence, France
pierrick.coupe@labri.fr
[2] Univ. Bordeaux, LaBRI, UMR 5800, PICTURA, 33400 Talence, France
[3] Neurocentre Magendie, INSERM U1215, 33077 Bordeaux, France
[4] Univ. Bordeaux, 33000 Bordeaux, France
[5] CHU de Bordeaux, Services de Neurologie et Neuroradiologie,
Bordeaux, France
[6] Instituto de Aplicaciones de las Tecnologías de la Información y de las
Comunicaciones Avanzadas (ITACA), Universitat Politècnica de València,
Camino de Vera s/n, 46022 Valencia, Spain

Abstract. In this paper, we present a new tool for white matter lesion segmentation called lesionBrain. Our method is based on a 3-stage strategy including multimodal patch-based segmentation, patch-based regularization of probability map and patch-based error correction using an ensemble of shallow neural networks. Its robustness and accuracy have been evaluated on the MSSEG challenge 2016 datasets. During our validation, the performance obtained by lesionBrain was competitive compared to recent deep learning methods. Moreover, lesionBrain proposes automatic lesion categorization according to location. Finally, complementary information on gray matter atrophy is included in the generated report. LesionBrain follows *a software as a service* model in full open access.

Keywords: White matter lesion segmentation · Patch-based segmentation
Service as a software

1 Introduction

The presence of white matter lesions (WML) is associated with different brain diseases such as multiple sclerosis (MS), small vessel disease or head injury among others, but it also occurs in normal aging. Magnetic resonance imaging (MRI), especially FLAIR images, has been found to be very sensitive in the detection of these WML. Therefore, MRI is the reference standard to identify WML and it plays a crucial role in the diagnosis and the monitoring of many neurological pathologies. Despite the importance of quantifying WML, this task remains mainly based on manual counting of lesions or semi quantitative scores such as Fazekas score. Manual delineation for volumetric analyses is extremely time-consuming and prone to errors due to inter- and intra-rater variability. As a result, the automation of WML segmentation has received a great deal

© Springer Nature Switzerland AG 2018
W. Bai et al. (Eds.): Patch-MI 2018, LNCS 11075, pp. 95–103, 2018.
https://doi.org/10.1007/978-3-030-00500-9_11

of attention during the last decade and a wide range of methods have been proposed [1]. These methods are usually classified into two categories, unsupervised and supervised. Unsupervised methods do not require a training dataset with manual segmentation of the lesions. These methods estimate lesions mainly using MRI intensities and some anatomical knowledge. They can be based on Bayesian models, Graph-cut [2] or thresholding approaches [3] among others. Supervised methods require a training dataset including manual segmentations of experts to learn from examples. Many different techniques have been proposed such as Random Forest [4], Patch-based methods [5, 6] and more recently deep learning methods [7–9]. Although automatic methods are becoming more and more accurate, manual segmentation remains used especially in clinical research or clinical trials in which very accurate quantification is needed to use lesion load as judgement criteria. Several factors can explain the difficulty to apply automatic methods in clinical context.

First, validating the accuracy of WML segmentation methods is challenging because of the difficulty to define a ground truth. Indeed, the high intra and inter-rater variability makes difficult to define a gold standard. Moreover, the lack of freely available annotated datasets leads to highly heterogeneous validation in the literature making methods comparison arduous. Therefore, it is difficult to appreciate the respective performances of automatic methods and their potential under clinical conditions. Recently, important efforts have been done to limit these aspects by sharing freely available datasets based on the consensus of several experts [10]. As a result, evaluation and comparison of methods become easier and more reliable. In this paper, we propose a new tool called lesionBrain which is an extension of the rotationally-invariant nonlocal means (RI-NLM) segmentation method [5]. To evaluate its performance compared to state-of-the-art methods, the validation is carried out on the MSSEG MICCAI Challenge 2016 dataset which is freely available providing a high quality ground truth based on the consensus of seven experts.

Second, few methods are freely available making their use in clinic research difficult. When available, these methods are usually distributed as packages that need to be downloaded, installed and configured. Installation steps can be complicated and thus may require experimented persons not always available in a research laboratory and especially in clinical context. In addition, users have to be trained to use the software and computational resources have to be allocated to run it. These requirements can make the use of these packages complex, especially the most recent and sophisticated ones requiring advanced hardware configuration (e.g., advanced GPU). To address this issue, lesionBrain is proposed as an online open access solution following the model of Software as a Service (SaaS). Our method works remotely through a web-interface and does not require any installation, resources or human interaction.

In addition, automatic methods generally provide the volume of WML as the sole output. However, complementary information can be relevant from a clinical point of view. Indeed, the location of lesions is useful to establish a diagnosis of multiple sclerosis after a first clinical episode according to the McDonald diagnosis criteria for MS [11]. To provide this information, lesionBrain proposes a lesion classification based on their proximity to lateral ventricles, cerebral cortex or cerebellum and brain stem. As a result, the lesion load in volume and also the number of lesions are provided for periventricular, juxtacortical, infratentorial and deep white matter areas.

Finally, most of the existing tools provide information focused on WML. However, complementary information from other structures might be needed to better study brain pathologies globally. For instance, gray matter (GM) atrophy can provide relevant information to investigate the neurodegenerative impact of MS or Alzheimer's Disease (AD). Therefore, lesionBrain not only provides volumetric measurement on WML but also a quantification of WM, GM and Cerebrospinal fluid (CSF). When age and gender of the subject are available, the volumes of these brain tissues are compared to reference values derived from lifespan models to detect abnormalities [12].

2   Materials and Methods

2.1   Datasets

LesionBrain Dataset: Our training dataset is composed of 43 patients who underwent 3T 3D-T1w MPRAGE and 3D-Fluid-Attenuated Inversion Recovery (FLAIR) MRI. The preprocessing steps described in the next subsection have been applied to all the images to align them into the MNI space and to normalize their intensities. Afterwards, a first expert performed manual segmentations in the MNI space for all the patients with ITKsnap [13] using T1w and FLAIR images. Then, a second expert validated and/or corrected all the manual segmentations. At the end, all the images were flipped as done in [14] to double the size of our training library (i.e., 86 training images).

MSSEG MICCAI Challenge 2016 Dataset: To evaluate our tools, we used the dataset of the MSSEG MICCAI Challenge 2016 [10]. For this dataset, 15 patients underwent 3D-T1w MPRAGE, 3D-FLAIR, Gadolinium- enhanced T1w, Proton Density (PD), and T2w MRI. Only T1w and FLAIR MRI were used during our experiments. These 15 subjects consist in 3 groups of five subjects scanned with Philips Ingenia 3T, Siemens Aera 1.5T and Siemens Verio 3T. All the images have been manually delineated by seven experts. Finally, the experts' consensus is used as gold standard.

2.2   Pipeline Description

Preprocessing: First, the images are preprocessed to normalize their intensity and to register them into the MNI space. A denoising step based on the adaptive nonlocal means filter is first applied to T1w and FLAIR images [15]. Both denoised MRI are then coarsely corrected for inhomogeneity [16]. Afterwards, the T1w is registered into the MNI space using an affine transform [17]. FLAIR is then registered to T1w in the MNI space. A fine inhomogeneity correction is performed on both images [18]. Finally, brain tissue maps (i.e., WM, GM and CSF) are obtained using [19]. These tissue maps are used to perform intensity normalization based on a piece-wise linear scaling of intensity where the median intensity of each tissue is set to a fixed value [20].

Structure Segmentation: The T1w is used to segment several anatomical structures. First, the intracranial cavity (ICC) is extracted using [21] and brainstem and cerebellum using [22]. Finally, lateral ventricles are segmented using [23].

Candidate Map: To reduce computational time, the segmentation is performed only on areas which potentially contain lesions as defined below. As done in [4, 6], the mean μ and the standard deviation σ of the GM FLAIR intensities are used to estimate a threshold (th $= \mu + \alpha\sigma$, with $\alpha = 0.5$). All voxels above this threshold and within the ICC mask are considered as lesion candidates. However, FLAIR intensity within lesion may sometimes be below this threshold. Therefore, an atlas of lesions (average of all the manual lesion maps of the lesionBrain dataset in the MNI space) is also used to look for lesions at the most probable location. Voxels at locations with probability higher than 20% to contain a lesion are added to the map of candidates obtained by thresholding.

Lesions Segmentation: Lesions are segmented using an extension of the RI-NLM method proposed in [5]. On the one hand, such voxel-wise method may produce false positive detections especially in cortical areas while implicit regularization of multipoint/patch-wise frameworks demonstrated better performance than voxel-wise approaches [20]. On the other hand, using patch-wise methods for lesion segmentation does not enable to efficiently capture heterogeneity of shape, size and location of lesions [5]. Therefore, in lesionBrain, we propose to apply first the RI-NLM method on T1w and FLAIR images to obtain the probability map of lesions. Second, we achieve a regularization of the probability map using a patch-wise NLM denoising filter [24]. The weights of the NLM filter are estimated on the FLAIR and then used to average the probabilities. The RI-NLM takes advantage of inter-subject similarity while patch-wise NLM regularization (NLMr) takes advantage of intra-subject similarity. Finally, a systematic error correction step is performed to obtain the final segmentation. Automatic correction of systematic errors was first proposed in [25] with SegAdapter. In lesionBrain, we used the Patch-based Ensemble Corrector (PEC) proposed in [26]. Contrary to SegAdapter which is based on a voxel-wise Adaboost classifier, PEC involves patch-wise ensemble of multilayer perceptron classifiers. Recently, second-pass strategy such as cascade of Convolutional Neural Networks (CNN) [9] demonstrated high performance to limit false positive detection.

Lesions Classification: Once the lesions are segmented, a last step is performed to classify them into the following categories: periventricular, juxtacortical, deep white and infratentorial. Such classification might be clinically relevant since some diagnose criteria of MS are based on it [11]. Therefore, all the lesions located within 3 voxels (i.e., 3 mm in the MNI space) from the lateral ventricles, the GM map, and the union of brainstem and cerebellum are classified respectively as periventricular, juxtacortical and infratentorial. The remaining lesions located in WM map are classified as deep white.

Report Generation: At the end, a pdf report is automatically generated providing the lesion load, the number of lesions for each class and screenshots of the processed images. Moreover, in case the gender and the age of the patient are provided, the estimated volumes of WM, GM and CSF are compared to expected normal values based on lifespan models [12]. The proposed lesionBrain tool has been integrated into the volBrain[1] platform in full open access [20].

2.3   Validation Framework

First, the method parameters were validated using training lesionBrain dataset through a K-fold cross validation. For RI-NLM segmentation and NLMr of the probability map, the patch size was set to $3 \times 3 \times 3$ voxels as proposed in the original papers [5, 24]. The search area was set to $9 \times 9 \times 9$ voxels for RI-NLM and NLMr although $11 \times 11 \times 11$ voxels is suggested in [5, 24]. This enables to reduce computational time with marginal accuracy loss. The number of used training images was set to the maximum (i.e., 86 when testing on the MSSEG Challenge 2016 dataset). For PEC we used the default parameters [26]. Therefore, the number of networks was set to 10 and the two patch scales to $3 \times 3 \times 3$ voxels and $7 \times 7 \times 7$ voxels. During the validation, we first evaluate the improvement in terms of mean DICE coefficient provided by each component of the proposed segmentation pipeline – RI-NLM, RI-NLM + NLMr and RI-NLM + NLMr + PEC (i.e., lesionBrain). Then, lesionBrain is compared with six state-of-the-art methods. To this end, we used the mean DICE coefficient published by authors who have evaluated their method on the 15 MS patients of the training MSSEG Challenge 2016 dataset as we did here. First, lesionBrain is compared with two unsupervised methods based on graph-cut [2] and thresholding as implemented in LST-LPA [3]. In addition, the proposed method is compared with four supervised methods including Random Forest [4] and recent advanced DL methods such as U-Net [7], Nabla-Net [8] and Dense-Net [7]. Finally, the inter-expert variability estimated in [4] between the seven experts is provided for reference purposes.

3   Results

First, Table 1 presents the mean DICE coefficient obtained with RI-NLM, RI-NLM + NLMr and lesionBrain of the MSSEG Challenge 2016 dataset. These results show that each component of the pipeline improved the segmentation accuracy. The mean DICE increased from 66.59% to 69.27% with the NLMr of the probability map and from 69.27% to 72.49% with PEC. Both improvements were found to be significant when tested with a paired t-test. This demonstrates the advantage of combining methods based on inter-subject similarity, intra-subject self-similarity and correction of systematic errors. Table 1 also shows the comparison of lesionBrain with six state-of-the-art methods. First, lesionBrain obtained the best mean DICE coefficient with 72.49 followed by the Dense-Net proposed in [24] which obtained 70.30. It has to be noted that lesionBrain only requires 2 contrasts while Dense-Net uses 5 contrasts. Increasing the number of sequences has a negative impact on the acquisition time, the patient's comfort and the related costs. In addition, the Dense-Net has been trained using cross-validation which can introduce overfitting and thus overestimates the performance of

---

[1] http://volbrain.upv.es

Table 1. Methods comparison on the 15 MS patients of the MSSEG challenge 2016 dataset in term of mean DICE coefficient.

Methods	Mean DICE in %	Training	Modalities
Inter-expert variability [4]	63.02		
lesionBrain	72.49	External	T1w and FLAIR
Dense-Net [7]	70.30	Cross-validation	T1, T1Gd, T2, PD and FLAIR
RI-NLM [5] + NLMr	69.27	External	T1w and FLAIR
Nabla-Net [8]	67.00	External	FLAIR
RI-NLM [5]	66.59	External	T1w and FLAIR
Random Forest [4]	63.80	Cross-validation	T1w and FLAIR
LST-LPA [3]	61.00	Unsupervised	FLAIR
Graph-cut [2]	57.09	Unsupervised	T1, T2 and FLAIR
U-Net [7]	56.42	Cross-validation	T1, T1Gd, T2, PD and FLAIR

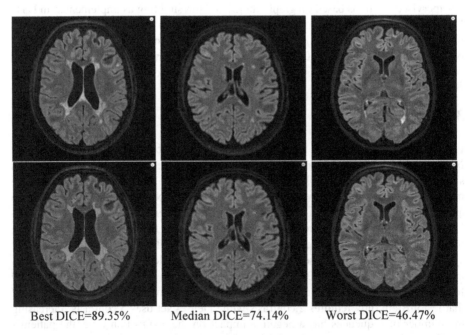

Best DICE=89.35%   Median DICE=74.14%   Worst DICE=46.47%

Fig. 1. Examples of WML segmentation produced by lesionBrain for best, median and worst DICE obtained on the MSSEG Challenge 2016 dataset. True positives are in green, False Negatives in red and False Positives in blue. (Color figure online)

the method. The Nabla-Net proposed in [8] requires only one contrast and has been trained on external dataset. This method obtained a DICE of 67% which is similar to the accuracy obtained by RI-NLM with 2 contrasts, but less than the accuracy obtained with RI-NLM + NLMr or lesionBrain.

Compared to Random Forest [4] which obtained 63.80% of accuracy, RI-NLM, RI-NLM + NLMr and lesionBrain obtained higher accuracy while they require the same contrasts. All these methods obtained accuracy higher than inter-expert variability estimated at 63.02% contrary to the 3 remaining ones. The two unsupervised methods based on graph-cut [3] and LST-LPA [3] obtained a mean DICE of 57.09% and 61% respectively. Finally, the U-Net method proposed in [7] obtained the worst accuracy with 56.42%. These results indicate that supervised methods are ranked among the best, better than inter-expert variability, while unsupervised methods failed to reach inter-expert variability. However, the use of CNN does not necessarily ensure a good accuracy since the worst method is based on a U-Net using 5 contrasts. Finally, Fig. 1 shows examples of WML segmentation obtained by lesionBrain for three patients of the MSSEG Challenge 2016 dataset (for best, median and worst DICE).

4 Conclusion

In this paper, we present a new tool for WML segmentation using T1w and FLAIR MRI. Our method combined several complementary patch-based approaches to accurately segment WML. We evaluated its accuracy on the MSSEG challenge 2016 datasets with a strong ground truth based on the consensus of seven experts. During our validation, the performance obtained by lesionBrain were competitive compared to Dense-Net [7], Nabla-Net [8] and U-Net [7]. Moreover, lesionBrain obtained a higher accuracy than the inter-expert variability. Finally, our tool is already integrated into a web-platform in open access.

Acknowledgement. This work benefited from the support of the project DeepVolBrain of the French National Research Agency (ANR). This study was achieved within the context of the Laboratory of Excellence TRAIL ANR-10-LABX-57 for the BigDataBrain project. Moreover, we thank the Investments for the future Program IdEx Bordeaux (ANR-10-IDEX- 03- 02, HL-MRI Project), Cluster of excellence CPU and the CNRS. This study has been also supported by the DPI2017-87743-R grant from the Spanish Ministerio de Economia, Industria y Competitividad.

References

1. Garcia-Lorenzo, D., et al.: Review of automatic segmentation methods of multiple sclerosis white matter lesions on conventional magnetic resonance imaging. Med. Image Anal. **17**(1), 1–18 (2013)
2. Beaumont, J., Commowick, O., Barillot, C.: Multiple Sclerosis lesion segmentation using an automated multimodal Graph Cut (2016)
3. Schmidt, P., et al.: An automated tool for detection of FLAIR-hyperintense white-matter lesions in multiple sclerosis. Neuroimage **59**(4), 3774–3783 (2012)

4. Vera-Olmos, F.J., Melero, H., Malpica, N.: Random forest for multiple sclerosis lesion segmentation. In: MSSEG Challenge Proceedings: Multiple Sclerosis Lesions Segmentation Challenge Using a Data Management and Processing Infrastructure, p. 81 (2016)
5. Guizard, N., et al.: Rotation-invariant multi-contrast non-local means for MS lesion segmentation. Neuroimage Clin. **8**, 376–389 (2015)
6. Mechrez, R., Goldberger, J., Greenspan, H.: Patch-based segmentation with spatial consistency: application to MS lesions in brain MRI. J. Biomed. Imaging **2016**, 1687–4188 (2016)
7. Hashemi, S.R., et al.: Tversky as a Loss Function for Highly Unbalanced Image Segmentation using 3D Fully Convolutional Deep Networks. arXiv preprint arXiv:1803.11078 (2018)
8. McKinley, R., et al.: Nabla-net: a deep dag-like convolutional architecture for biomedical image segmentation: application to white-matter lesion segmentation in multiple sclerosis. In: MSSEG Challenge Proceedings: Multiple Sclerosis Lesions Segmentation Challenge Using a Data Management and Processing Infrastructure, p. 37 (2016)
9. Valverde, S., et al.: Improving automated multiple sclerosis lesion segmentation with a cascaded 3D convolutional neural network approach. NeuroImage **155**, 159–168 (2017)
10. Commowick, O., Cervenansky, F., Ameli, R.: MSSEG Challenge Proceedings: Multiple Sclerosis Lesions Segmentation Challenge Using a Data Management and Processing Infrastructure (2016)
11. Thompson, A.J., et al.: Diagnosis of multiple sclerosis: 2017 revisions of the McDonald criteria. In: The Lancet Neurology, pp. 1474–4422 (2017)
12. Coupe, P., et al.: Towards a unified analysis of brain maturation and aging across the entire lifespan: a MRI analysis. Hum. Brain Mapp. **38**(11), 5501–5518 (2017)
13. Yushkevich, P.A., et al.: User-guided 3D active contour segmentation of anatomical structures: significantly improved efficiency and reliability. Neuroimage **31**(3), 1116–1128 (2006)
14. Eskildsen, S.F., et al.: BEaST: brain extraction based on nonlocal segmentation technique. Neuroimage **59**(3), 2362–2373 (2012)
15. Manjon, J.V., et al.: Adaptive non-local means denoising of MR images with spatially varying noise levels. J. Magn. Reson. Imaging **31**(1), 192–203 (2010)
16. Tustison, N.J., et al.: N4ITK: improved N3 bias correction. IEEE Trans. Med. Imaging **29**(6), 1310–1320 (2010)
17. Avants, B.B., et al.: A reproducible evaluation of ANTs similarity metric performance in brain image registration. Neuroimage **54**(3), 2033–2044 (2011)
18. Weiskopf, N., et al.: Unified segmentation based correction of R1 brain maps for RF transmit field inhomogeneities (UNICORT). Neuroimage **54**(3), 2116–2124 (2011)
19. Manjón, J.V., Tohka, J., Robles, M.: Improved estimates of partial volume coefficients from noisy brain MRI using spatial context. Neuroimage **53**(2), 480–490 (2010)
20. Manjon, J.V., Coupe, P.: volBrain: an online MRI brain volumetry system. Front. Neuroinform. **10**, 30 (2016)
21. Manjon, J.V., et al.: Nonlocal intracranial cavity extraction. Int. J. Biomed. Imaging **2014**, 820205 (2014)
22. Romero, J.E., et al.: NABS: non-local automatic brain hemisphere segmentation. Magn. Reason. Imaging **33**(4), 474–484 (2015)
23. Coupé, P., et al.: Patch-based segmentation using expert priors: application to hippocampus and ventricle segmentation. Neuroimage **54**(2), 940–954 (2011)
24. Coupe, P., et al.: An optimized blockwise nonlocal means denoising filter for 3-D magnetic resonance images. IEEE Trans. Med. Imaging **27**(4), 425–441 (2008)

25. Wang, H., et al.: A learning-based wrapper method to correct systematic errors in automatic image segmentation: consistently improved performance in hippocampus, cortex and brain segmentation. Neuroimage **55**(3), 968–985 (2011)

26. Romero, J.E., Coupé, P., Manjón, J.V.: HIPS: a new hippocampus subfield segmentation method. NeuroImage **163**, 286–295 (2017)

Multi-atlas Parcellation in the Presence of Lesions: Application to Multiple Sclerosis

Sandra González-Villà[1,2]([⊠]), Yuankai Huo[2], Arnau Oliver[1], Xavier Lladó[1], and Bennett A. Landman[2]

[1] Institute of Computer Vision and Robotics, University of Girona, Ed. P-IV, Campus Montilivi, 17003 Girona, Spain
`sgonzalez@eia.udg.edu`
[2] Electrical Engineering, Vanderbilt University, Nashville, TN 37235, USA

Abstract. Intensity-based multi-atlas strategies have shown leading performance in segmenting healthy subjects, but when lesions are present, the abnormal lesion intensities affect the fusion result. Here, we propose a reformulated statistical fusion approach for multi-atlas segmentation that is applicable to both healthy and injured brains. This method avoids the interference of lesion intensities on the segmentation by incorporating two *a priori* masks to the Non-Local STAPLE statistical framework. First, we extend the theory to include a lesion mask, which improves the voxel correspondence between the target and the atlases. Second, we extend the theory to include a known label mask, that forces the label decision in case it is beforehand known and enables seamless integration of manual edits. We evaluate our method with simulated and MS patient images and compare our results with those of other state-of-the-art multi-atlas strategies: Majority vote, Non-local STAPLE, Non-local Spatial STAPLE and Joint Label Fusion. Quantitative and qualitative results demonstrate the improvement in the lesion areas.

Keywords: Brain parcellation · Segmentation · Multiple sclerosis

1 Introduction

Brain parcellation has become an essential tool for understanding neurological structural-functional associations at a millimeter scale. The resulting voxelwise tissue classifications are integral to identifying structural regions for connectomics, functional activations, quantitative/metabolical changes, diffusion connectivity, etcetera. These techniques require reproducible segmentations; however, manual delineation is time-consuming, exhibits poor reproducibility, and is subject to inter- and intra- operator variability. For these reasons, automatic brain parcellation has been widely studied [1–3]. Several automatic strategies have been proposed in the literature to segment brain structures, such as deformable, learning-based, region-based, etc. [4–6]; however, most of these

© Springer Nature Switzerland AG 2018
W. Bai et al. (Eds.): Patch-MI 2018, LNCS 11075, pp. 104–113, 2018.
https://doi.org/10.1007/978-3-030-00500-9_12

methods are structure-specific and do not allow segmentation of the whole brain. In contrast, atlas-based strategies provide a whole parcellation when the atlases used have all the structures labelled.

In multi-atlas segmentation, a collection of atlases is registered to the target image and their labels are propagated and fused in the target image space, obtaining the final segmentation. Label fusion strategies based on intensities [7–10] have been demonstrated to be robust and provide good performance when dealing with healthy subjects. However, as most other state-of-the-art methods, they are designed to segment healthy subjects and their performance tends to be affected when segmenting brains hindered by tumors and lesions, for instance, as a result of multiple sclerosis (MS) [12].

Herein, we propose a novel statistical fusion algorithm that reformulates the non-local STAPLE (NLS) [8] statistical framework to handle (anatomical) MRI visible lesions. As in NLS, our method models the registered atlases as collections of volumetric patches with intensity and label information. To complement the non-local criteria, we introduce lesion mask information to resolve the imperfect correspondences between the healthy atlases and the lesioned target derived from inaccurate registrations. Additionally, a second mask is integrated into the estimation process, which forces the voxel label assignation in case it is known beforehand. For instance, this modification is useful when segmenting brains with tumors for which sub-regions are known. Together, these innovations enable inclusion of masks of abnormal anatomy and manually provided *edits* within modern statistical fusion approaches. We derive the theoretical basis governing our method and demonstrate segmentation improvement with respect to other multi-atlas strategies on the state of the art on both simulated and MS images.

2   Theory

Consider a target gray-level image (with lesions) represented as a vector $I \in \mathbb{R}^{N \times 1}$. Let $T \in \mathcal{L}^{N \times 1}$ be the latent representation of the true target segmentation, where $\mathcal{L} = \{0, \ldots, L-1\}$ is the set of possible labels which can be assigned to a concrete voxel. Let $M \in \{0, 1\}^{N \times 1}$ be a binary lesion mask indicating whether a given voxel i of the target image contains or is part of a lesion and $K \in \{0, 1\}^{N \times 1}$ a second mask specifying if for a given voxel i of the target image, the true label is known, hence $M_i = p(I_i \in lesion)$ and $K_i = p(T_i = T_k \in \mathcal{L}^{N \times 1})$. Note that both masks are optional and can be neglected if all voxels in the mask are set to 0. Consider a set R of registered healthy atlases with associated gray level images, $A \in \mathbb{R}^{N \times R}$, and propagated label decisions, $D \in \mathcal{L}^{N \times R}$. Let $\theta \in [0, 1]^{R \times N \times L \times L}$ be the performance level parameters of the raters (registered atlases), defined voxel-wise. Each element of θ, $\theta_{jis's}$, represents the probability that rater j observes label s' given that the true label is s at a given voxel i and the corresponding voxel i^* on the associated atlas—i.e., $\theta_{jis's} = p(D_{i^*j} = s', A_j | T_i = s, I_i, M_i, K_i, \theta_{jis's})$, where i^* is the voxel on atlas j that corresponds to the target voxel i.

2.1   Non-local Correspondence Model

Non-local STAPLE (NLS) [8] incorporates the concept of patch-based non-local correspondence based on the image intensities of both the target image I and the registered atlases A to the STAPLE framework. Although this concept has proven useful for matching healthy tissues to account for registration accuracy, we cannot rely on intensity similarities between the target lesion areas and the healthy atlases to rectify registration errors. Therefore, we assume that voxel correspondence inside the lesions cannot be further improved based on intensity and, hence, enforce the non-local weighting ($\alpha_{ji'i}$) between voxel i in the target image at voxel i' on the jth atlas as follows:

$$\alpha_{ji'i} = \left(\frac{1}{Z_\alpha} \exp \left(-\frac{\|\wp_{M_i} \circ (\wp(A_{i'j}) - \wp(I_i))\|_2^2}{2 \cdot \sigma_i^2 \cdot \|\wp_{M_i}\|} \right) \exp \left(-\frac{\varepsilon_{i'i}^2}{2 \cdot \sigma_d^2} \right) \right) \cdot (1 - M_i) \\ + \delta (i' = i) \cdot M_i \tag{1}$$

where $\wp(\cdot)$ is the set of intensities in the patch neighborhood of a given intensity location. In this definition, $\wp_{M_i} = \wp(1 - M_i)$ is the masking term that excludes lesion voxels from the patch calculation and enforces the same patch neighborhood size/shape in both the atlas and the target, $\|\wp_{M_i} \circ (\wp(A_{i'j} - \wp(I_i))\|_2^2$ is the L2-norm between the atlas patch centered at i' and the target patch centered at i, $\varepsilon_{i'i}^2$ is the Euclidean distance in physical space between i and i', σ_i and σ_d are the standard deviations of the intensity and distance weights, and Z_α is a partition function that enforces the constraint that $\sum_{i' \in \mathcal{N}(i)} \alpha_{ji'i} = 1$, where $\mathcal{N}(i)$ is the set of voxels in the search neighborhood of a given target voxel. $\delta(i' = i)$ is the Dirac delta function, and $\|\wp_{M_i}\|$ is the number of voxels in the patch neighborhood.

2.2   The Algorithm

If the exact voxel correspondences between the target and the atlases (non-local model) were known, the lesion mask, and the target and atlas intensity relationships could be ignored and the spatial STAPLE [11] definition of θ could be used.

$$\theta_{jis's} \equiv p(D_{i*j} = s', A_j | T_i = s, I_i, M_i, K_i, \theta_{jis's}) \\ = p(D_{i*j} = s' | T_i = s, M_i, K_i, \theta_{jis's}) \tag{2}$$

However, this correspondence is not known and we have to learn it with the model defined in Sect. 2.1. Note that using this model we can approximate the relationship by taking the expected value of $p(D_{i*j} = s', A_j | T_i = s, I_i, M_i, K_i, \theta_{jis's})$ across the raters. Using an assumption of conditional independence between the labels, lesion mask and intensity, we approximate the density function as:

$$p(D_{i*j} = s', A_j | T_i = s, I_i, M_i, K_i, \theta_{jis's}) \approx E[p(D_j, A_j | T_i = s, I_i, M_i, K_i, \theta_{jis})] \\ = E[p(D_j | T_i = s, M_i, K_i, \theta_{jis}) \cdot p(A_j | I_i, M_i)] \\ = \sum_{i' \in \mathcal{N}(i)} p(D_{i*j} = s' | T_i = s, M_i, K_i, \theta_{jis's}) \cdot p(A_{i'j} | I_i, M_i) = \sum_{i' \in \mathcal{N}(i)} \theta_{jis's} \cdot \alpha_{ji'i} \tag{3}$$

E-step. Let $W \in \mathbb{R}^{L \times N}$, where $W_{si}^{(t)}$ represents the probability that the true label associated with voxel i is s at iteration t of the algorithm given the provided information and the performance level parameters.

$$W_{si}^{(t)} \equiv p\left(T_i = s | D, A, I, M, K, \theta^{(t)}\right) \tag{4}$$

Using Bayes' rule to separate the prior label probability ($p(T_i = s)$) and assuming independence among the raters, we can rewrite this equation as follows:

$$W_{si}^{(t)} \equiv \frac{(1-K_i)\cdot\left(p(T_i=s)\cdot\prod_j p\left(D_{i*j}=s',A_j|T_i=s,I_i,M_i,K_i,\theta_{jis's}^{(t)}\right)\right)+K_i\cdot\delta(s'=s)}{(1-K_i)\cdot\left(\sum_n p(T_i=n)\cdot\prod_j p\left(D_{i*j}=s',A_j|T_i=n,I_i,M_i,K_i,\theta_{jis's}^{(t)}\right)\right)+K_i\cdot\delta(s'=s)} \tag{5}$$

where $\delta(s'=s)$ is the Dirac delta function (probability that the known label for voxel i of the truth segmentation is s). Using the non-local correspondence model and the approximated density function, we obtain:

$$W_{si}^{(t)} \equiv \frac{(1-K_i)\cdot\left(p(T_i=s)\cdot\prod_j \sum_{i'\in\mathcal{N}(i)} \theta_{jis's}^{(t)}\cdot\alpha_{ji'i}\right)+K_i\cdot\delta(s'=s)}{(1-K_i)\cdot\left(\sum_n p(T_i=n)\cdot\prod_j \sum_{i'\in\mathcal{N}(i)} \theta_{jis's}^{(t)}\cdot\alpha_{ji'i}\right)+K_i\cdot\delta(s'=s)} \tag{6}$$

M-step. In this step, the calculated $W_{si}^{(t)}$ is used to update $\theta_{ji}^{(t+1)}$ by maximizing the expectation of the complete data log likelihood. As the complete data log likelihood is not observable, it is replaced by its conditional expectation given the observable data D, A, I, M, K using the current estimate θ.

$$\theta_{ji}^{(t+1)} = \arg\max_{\theta_{ji}} \sum_{i'\in\mathcal{B}_i} E\left[\ln\left(p\left(D_j, A_j|T_{i'}, I_{i'}, M_{i'}, K_{i'}, \theta_{ji}|D, A, I, M, K, \theta^{(t)}\right)\right)\right]$$

$$= \arg\max_{\theta_{ji}} \sum_{i'\in\mathcal{B}_i} \sum_s p\left(T_{i'} = s|D, A, I, M, K, \theta^{(t)}\right) \cdot \ln\left(p\left(D_j, A_j|T_{i'}, I_{i'}, M_{i'}, K_{i'}, \theta_{ji}\right)\right)$$

$$= \arg\max_{\theta_{ji}} \sum_{i'\in\mathcal{B}_i} \sum_s W_{si'}^{(t)} \cdot \ln\left(p\left(D_{i*j} = s', A_j|T_{i'}, I_{i'}, M_{i'}, K_{i'}, \theta_{ji}\right)\right)$$

$$= \arg\max_{\theta_{ji}} \sum_{i'\in\mathcal{B}_i} \sum_s W_{si'}^{(t)} \cdot \ln\left(\sum_{i''\in\mathcal{N}(i'):D_{i''j}=s'} \theta_{jis's} \cdot \alpha_{ji''i'}\right) \tag{7}$$

As each row of θ must sum one to be a valid probability mass function, we can maximize the performance level parameters for each element by using a Lagrange multiplier (λ) to formulate the constrained optimization problem.

$$0 = \frac{\delta}{\delta\theta_{jin'n}}\left[\sum_{i'\in\mathcal{B}_i} \sum_s W_{si'}^{(t)} \cdot \ln\left(\sum_{i''\in\mathcal{N}(i'):D_{i''j}=s'} \theta_{jis's} \cdot \alpha_{ji''i'}\right) + \lambda\sum_{s'}\theta_{jis's}^{(t+1)}\right] \tag{8}$$

By solving this equation, we obtain

$$\theta_{jis's}^{(t+1)} = \frac{\sum_{i'\in\mathcal{B}_i}\left(\sum_{i''\in\mathcal{N}(i'):D_{i''j}=s'} \alpha_{ji''i'}\right) \cdot W_{si'}^{(t)}}{\sum_{i'\in\mathcal{B}_i} W_{si'}^{(t)}} \tag{9}$$

2.3   Initialization and Priors

The voxel-wise prior $p(T_i = s)$ was initialized using the weak log-odds majority vote, as in NLSS. The performance parameters, $\theta_{jis's}$, were initialized assuming each atlas has high performance as: 1, if $s = s'$; 0.95, if $s = s'$; 0, if $s \neq s'$; and $\frac{0.05}{L-1}$, otherwise. The search neighborhood $\mathcal{N}(\cdot)$ was set to $7 \times 7 \times 7$, patch $\wp(\cdot)$ dimensions to $5 \times 5 \times 5$ and σ_i and σ_d were set to 0.25 and 1.5, respectively. Algorithm convergence was detected when the average change in the diagonal elements of θ was below 10^{-4}.

3   Experiments and Results

The atlases used in our experiments were taken from the MICCAI 2012 Grand Challenge and Workshop on Multi-Atlas Labeling database [13]. This database consists of 35 T1-w MR images, obtained from the OASIS[1] project and labeled by Neuromorphometrics, Inc.[2], and includes labels for the whole brain. PCA atlas selection was performed and only the 15 most similar atlases were used for segmentation. All images were histogram normalized and N4 bias field corrected before registration. All pair-wise registrations were performed using an initial affine registration (niftyreg[3]) followed by a non-rigid (ANTs[4]) procedure. In all the registrations performed, the lesions were masked-out to avoid their intensities to interfere in the similarity metric calculation.

As benchmarks, we compare the proposed algorithm to majority vote (MV) [14], non-local STAPLE (NLS) [8], non-local Spatial STAPLE (NLSS) [9] and Joint Label Fusion (JLF) [10]. For a fair comparison, all the parameters that NLS and NLSS share with our algorithm were set to the same values. Also, JLF was executed with the same patch and neighborhood size.

3.1   Simulated Lesions

Evaluating the performance of segmentation algorithms on real lesioned images is not an easy task since there is a lack of public databases with ground truth for both lesions and structures. For this reason, in the first experiment, we simulated two sets of artificially lesioned images: (1) 10 with uniform intensity lesions, to test the proposed theory and, (2) 15 with lesion shapes, intensities and locations obtained from an in-house MS patient database, to simulate realistic cases. All the lesions were generated on random subjects from the MICCAI 2012 database. The lesion load of the generated images ranged from $[33.49-119.74]\,\mathrm{mm}^3$ in the first cohort and from $[3.16-26.96]\,\mathrm{mm}^3$ in the second one.

---

[1] http://www.oasis-brains.org/.

[2] http://neuromorphometrics.com/.

[3] http://cmictig.cs.ucl.ac.uk/wiki/index.php/NiftyReg.

[4] https://sourceforge.net/projects/advants/.

We evaluated the segmentation results quantitatively using a global Dice Similarity Coefficient (DSC) across all the structures as the main measure. As the lesion intensities not only necessarily affect the lesion area segmentation itself, but also the surrounding tissues, two measures were calculated: (1) DSC inside the lesion mask, and (2) DSC inside a mask that included three voxels of the contour. Note that $\mathcal{N}(\cdot)$ was set to $7 \times 7 \times 7$.

Figure 1(A) shows that, inside the lesion mask, our method performed significantly better than all the intensity-based strategies (JLF, NLS and NLSS) in both cohorts. However, the performance was similar to that of MV. This is due to the fact that we cannot trust the intensities inside the lesions, and we can only rely on an accurate registration (same as MV does). On the other hand, when the performance was analyzed around the lesion areas, our proposal was the one that provided the best results (similar to MV in the first cohort and to JLF in the second one). This behavior is depicted in Fig. 1(B), where JLF (b and h) misclassifies several structures inside the lesion areas, whereas in NLSS (c and i) the segmentation is being also affected in the surrounding structures.

For the evaluation of the manual edits (K mask integration), we segmented the first dataset again, this time feeding the algorithm with the same lesion mask for both M and K. The results showed, as expected, a DSC of 1 inside the lesion areas (M/K mask), whereas the mean DSC around the lesions was 0.7901 ± 0.0463, very similar to that of the first execution (0.7919 ± 0.0457), conserving a similar effect on the tissues surrounding the lesions.

3.2 MSSeg 2016 Challenge

For the second experiment, we qualitatively compared the fusion results obtained by the analyzed algorithms on a MS patient database (MSSeg 2016 challenge[5]).

Figure 2 shows the segmentations obtained with all the analyzed multi-atlas strategies. As we can observe from Fig. 2(a), MS lesions are hypo-intense in T1-w modality, which makes its intensity profile similar of that of the gray matter (GM) and even sometimes similar to the cerebro-spinal fluid (CSF) which may affect the results of intensity-based algorithms. The lesions shown in Fig. 2(b), should be classified as white matter, however, the intensity-based algorithms of the state of the art, Fig. 2(f–h), tend to misclassify those regions as GM or CSF, whereas our method, Fig. 2(c), shows better classification results in those areas. When our method is fed with a K mask, Fig. 2(d), the lesion surrounding voxels remain practically the same as when the K mask is not used, Fig. 2(c), whereas the segmentation result inside the lesions agrees entirely with the labels imposed by this mask, as seen in Sect. 3.1.

---

[5] https://portal.fli-iam.irisa.fr/msseg-challenge/overview.

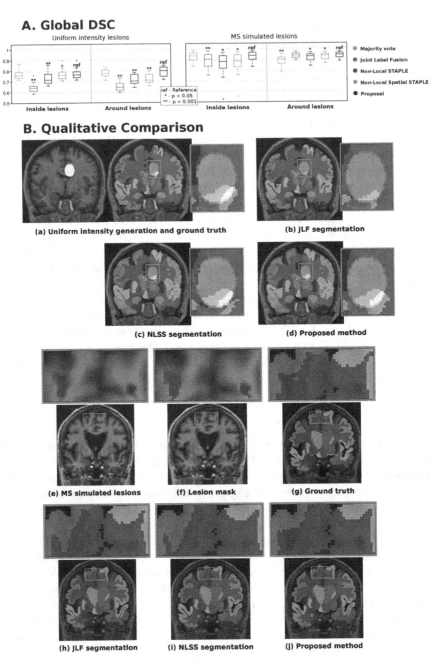

Fig. 1. (A) Global DSC and (B) qualitative segmentation results of analyzed multi-atlas strategies on both simulated databases: (a–d) uniform intensity lesions, and (e–j) MS simulated lesions.

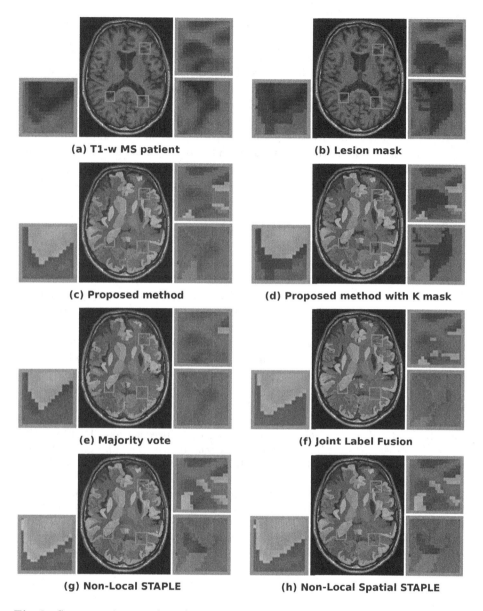

Fig. 2. Segmentation results of the analyzed multi-atlas strategies for the image 01038PAGU of the MICCAI2016 Challenge database.

4   Discussion

Accurate structural volume measurements are important in MS, since the atrophy of some structures such as the deep GM is relevant to the disease progression. However, we have shown that multi-atlas strategies based on intensities, which achieve good segmentation results on healthy subjects, are affected by lesions, and therefore corrupting real measures.

Herein, we have presented the theory to modify the non-local STAPLE framework to deal with MRI visible lesions. The experiments performed show that our proposal outperforms the state-of-the-art multi-atlas strategies in the lesion areas for both simulated and MS patient images.

Over-performance of MV compared to the state-of-the-art intensity-based strategies was observed on the experiments performed on the uniform intensity lesions database around the lesion areas. This behavior could be due to the fact that the other strategies are patch-based. These strategies consider mean patch differences to calculate the correspondences, hence the bright voxels of the lesions could bias the mean intensity, finding wrong atlas correspondences. Even though, this is an extreme case to test the proposed theory, it shows, combined with the over-performance of MV inside the lesion areas, the effect of the lesion intensities on the segmentation.

In this work, we have only focused on the segmentation performance of the lesion areas, since those are the ones concerning the proposed reformulation. Nonetheless, as these areas are better segmented with our strategy, the average whole brain segmentation performance slightly increases compared to the non-local STAPLE variants. This small improvement is due to lesions are small compared to the whole brain volume. For this reason, we believe that extending our theory to other methods of the literature, such as JLF, would be beneficial in terms of segmentation accuracy of the lesion areas but also of the whole brain.

Acknowledgements. The authors would like to thank Jose Bernal for helpful discussion. Sandra González-Villà holds a UdG-BRGR2015 grant. This work has been supported by "La Fundació la Marató de TV3", by Retos de Investigación TIN2014-55710-R and TIN2015-73563-JIN, by DPI2017-86696-R and by UdG mobility grant MOB17. This research was supported by NSF CAREER 1452485, NIH R01-EB017230, and the National Center for Advancing Translational Sciences, Grant 2 UL1 TR000445-06. We appreciate the NIH S10 Shared Instrumentation Grant 1S10OD020154-01 (Smith), Vanderbilt IDEAS grant (Holly-Bockelmann, Walker, Meliler, Palmeri, Weller), and ACCRE's Big Data TIPs grant from Vanderbilt University. The content is solely the responsibility of the authors and does not necessarily represent the official views of the National Institutes of Health, National Science Foundation, or other sponsors.

References

1. Iglesias, J.E., Sabuncu, M.R.: Multi-atlas segmentation of biomedical images: a survey. Med. Image Anal. **24**(1), 205–219 (2015)
2. Li, W., Wang, G., Fidon, L., Ourselin, S., Cardoso, M.J., Vercauteren, T.: On the compactness, efficiency, and representation of 3D convolutional networks: brain parcellation as a pretext task. In: Niethammer, M., et al. (eds.) IPMI 2017. LNCS, vol. 10265, pp. 348–360. Springer, Cham (2017). https://doi.org/10.1007/978-3-319-59050-9_28
3. Wachinger, C., Reuter, M., Klein, T.: DeepNAT: deep convolutional neural network for segmenting neuroanatomy. NeuroImage **170**, 434–445 (2018)

4. González-Villà, S., Oliver, A., Valverde, S., Wang, L., Zwiggelaar, R., Lladó, X.: A review on brain structures segmentation in magnetic resonance imaging. Artif. Intell. Med. **73**, 45–69 (2016)
5. Kushibar, K., et al.: Automated sub-cortical brain structure segmentation combining spatial and deep convolutional features. Med. Image Anal. **48**, 177–186 (2018)
6. Dolz, J., Desrosiers, C., Ayed, I.B.: 3D fully convolutional networks for subcortical segmentation in MRI: a large-scale study. NeuroImage **170**, 456–470 (2018)
7. Coupé, P., Manjón, J.V., Fonov, V., Pruessner, J., Robles, M., Collins, D.L.: Patch-based segmentation using expert priors: application to hippocampus and ventricle segmentation. NeuroImage **54**(2), 940–954 (2011)
8. Asman, A.J., Landman, B.A.: Non-local statistical label fusion for multi-atlas segmentation. Med. Image Anal. **17**(2), 194–208 (2013)
9. Huo, Y., Asman, A.J., Plassard, A.J., Landman, B.A.: Simultaneous total intracranial volume and posterior fossa volume estimation using multi-atlas label fusion. Hum. Brain Mapp. **38**(2), 599–616 (2017)
10. Wang, H., Suh, J.W., Das, S.R., Pluta, J.B., Craige, C., Yushkevich, P.A.: Multi-atlas segmentation with joint label fusion. IEEE Trans. Pattern Anal. Mach. Intell. **35**(3), 611–623 (2013)
11. Asman, A.J., Landman, B.A.: Formulating spatially varying performance in the statistical fusion framework. IEEE Trans. Med. Imaging **31**(6), 1326–1336 (2012)
12. González-Villà, S., et al.: Evaluating the effect of multiple sclerosis lesions on automatic brain structure segmentation. NeuroImage Clin. **15**, 228–238 (2017)
13. Landman, B., Warfield, S.: MICCAI 2012 workshop on multi-atlas labeling. In: MICCAI Grand Challenge and Workshop on Multi-Atlas Labeling, Nice, France (2012)
14. Sabuncu, M., Yeo, B., Van Leemput, K., Fischl, B., Golland, P.: A generative model for image segmentation based on label fusion. IEEE Trans. Med. Imaging **29**(10), 1714–1729 (2010)

A Patch-Based Segmentation Approach with High Level Representation of the Data for Cortical Sulci Recognition

Léonie Borne[(✉)], Jean-François Mangin, and Denis Rivière

Neurospin, CEA Saclay, 91191 Gif-sur-Yvette, France
leonie.borne@cea.fr

Abstract. Because of the strong variability of the cortical sulci, their automatic recognition is still a challenging problem. The last algorithm developed in our laboratory for 125 sulci reaches an average recognition rate around 86%. It has been applied to thousands of brains for morphometric studies (www.brainvisa.info). A weak point of this approach is the modeling of the training dataset as a single template of sulcus-wise probability maps, losing information about the alternative patterns of each sulcus. To overcome this limit, we propose a different strategy inspired by Multi-Atlas Segmentation (MAS) and more particularly the patch-based approaches. As the standard way of extracting patches does not seem capable of exploiting the sulci geometry and the relations between them, which we believe to be the discriminative features for recognition, we propose a new patch generation strategy based on a high level representation of the sulci. We show that our new approach is slightly, but significantly, better than the reference one, while we still have an avenue of potential refinements that were beyond reach for a single template strategy.

Keywords: MRI · Cortical sulci labeling · Patch-based segmentation

1 Introduction

1.1 Overview of Cortical Sulci Recognition Approaches

The surface of the human brain cortex is divided into gyri, separated by fissures called sulci. The largest sulci are good indicators of the localization of functional areas and the morphometry of the sulci geometry is used to quantify brain development and neurodegenerative processes. Automatic recognition is mandatory to exploit the large databases yielded by recent neuroimaging projects. However, automatic sulci recognition remains a challenging problem because of the lack of understanding of the nature of the interindividual variability of the folding patterns. During the last twenty years, many different approaches have been proposed to handle this problem.

© Springer Nature Switzerland AG 2018
W. Bai et al. (Eds.): Patch-MI 2018, LNCS 11075, pp. 114–121, 2018.
https://doi.org/10.1007/978-3-030-00500-9_13

The approaches based on atlas registration yield reasonable identification rate for major sulci. For instance, in [12], a labeled brain is elastically deformed to fit a new brain, and in [6], a multiresolution strategy is designed to improve the results by progressively registering the largest folds to the smallest folds. This **single template strategy however has strong limitations** with regard to the numerous folding configurations incompatible with the atlas geometry, which occurs even for the largest sulci.

Modeling intersubject variability seems mandatory to increase robustness, which was tackled using a variety of frameworks ranging from PCA to Bayesian approaches [1,5,7,9]. A large amount of strategies rely on graph-based representations, which provide a flexible way to model the spatial relationships between the sulci in addition to their shape and localization in a normalized space [3,10,11,13–15]. **Comparing these approaches is difficult in the absence of benchmark.** Furthermore, all of them except the one in BrainVISA are restricted to a small set of sulci, a small training database and are not distributed. Therefore, in this paper, we will only compare our new model to the results of BrainVISA current package.

1.2   The Current BrainVISA Model: Principles, Advantages and Inconvenients

The current BrainVISA model relies on a **coherent Bayesian framework** based on a probabilistic atlas (a model made of a mixture of Statistical Probabilistic Anatomy Maps (SPAM)). This approach performs simultaneously sulcus recognition and local alignment with the template of SPAMs [9]. Unfortunately, this approach performs poorly with unusual folding patterns, which depart from the main modes of the probabilistic atlas. This is a classical limitation of single template strategies. For instance, the reconfiguration of the folding patterns induced by interruptions of the large sulci can lead to inconsistent sulcus recognition. Furthermore, we have observed disturbing mistakes that did not occur with the older graph-based approach also proposed in BrainVISA [10]. For instance a large sulcus can be locally duplicated because the current Bayesian framework does not model the relationships between folds, while the previous graph-based approach could learn alternative configurations thanks to a neural network (NN) based memory. Unfortunately, this NN strategy could probably not be trained with a large enough manually labelled database to reach the robustness of the Bayesian framework.

1.3   MAS Strategy: A Solution to the Limits of the Current Model?

In biomedical image analysis, segmentation is the process of tagging image voxels with biologically meaningful labels. The MAS strategy has become one of the most widely-used and successful solution. The idea of this technique is to use for segmentation the entire dataset of "atlases" (i.e. training images) rather than one model-based average kind of representation, so that it better captures the anatomical variability. A power of this approach is its pragmatism: it can be applied for a problem where a real understanding of the nature of the interindividual variability is lacking, which fits the current status of the neuroscience world with regard to the cortical folding.

Most of the MAS techniques include four main steps: **(1) Atlas generation:** the design of atlases from the training images; **(2) Registration:** alignment of each atlas onto the new image to be segmented; **(3) Label propagation:** from each aligned atlas to the new subject, **(4) Label fusion:** combining the propagated labels to achieve the final segmentation. One of the most recent MAS techniques developed by Coupé et al. [4] performs a patch-based label fusion, which leads to very efficient implementations.

The problem of sulci recognition differs from standard MAS applications by several aspects. First, there are many more anatomical structures to be labeled: each brain contains up to 125 cortical sulci in the nomenclature of BrainVISA. Second and more importantly, grey level intensities and textures surrounding the sulci do not provide discriminative information except for a few sulci like central sulcus, because of a specific local myelin content. Therefore, the key discriminative information is folding geometry, which requires larger voxel-based patches than in usual implementations. Hence, for the sake of efficiency, in the following we will operate at a larger intermediate scale of representation of the folding patterns, where the entities to be labelled are predefined sets of voxels corresponding to the most elementary folds (about 500 such entities in a standard brain) [8].

The new model proposed in this article is inspired by the patch-based methodology proposed by Coupé et al. [4] but the patches are not defined as local groups of voxels but as local groups of sulci. Note that this strategy could be extended to all the domains where an **intermediate level of representation of the data** could be useful for the alignment of the atlases to the unknown subject. Hence, we have to revisit the different stages of the mainstream strategy to take into account the heterogeneity of the representations of the subjects. In the following, we design a dedicated patch generation strategy, a geometry-based measure of similarity to perform the patch-based alignment, and a propagation strategy for 3D points clouds.

2   Database

In order to compare our results to those of [9] in the same conditions, we use the exact same database of 62 healthy subjects selected from different heterogeneous databases. Most of the subjects are right-handed male persons, between 25 and 35 years old. The elementary folds of each brain were manually labelled according to the sulcus nomenclature following a long process leading to achieve a consensus across a set of several experts of the morphology of the cortex. Each fold representation is a set of voxels corresponding to the medial surface of the cerebrospinal fluid filling up the fold. Hence, these fold representations are elementary pieces of a negative mould of the brain. As mentioned above, the sulcus recognition method described in this paper will be forced to give one unique label to the set of voxels representing a fold. The training base is composed of 62 brains labelled with a model containing 62 sulci for the right hemisphere and 63 for the left.

3 Method: A New Model Inspired by MAS Algorithms

As the new model is inspired by the MAS strategy, the same steps are used and will be described in this section (Fig. 1). In the following, the atlas brains and the new brain are all represented as a set of elementary folds. All the atlas folds have been manually labelled with the sulcus nomenclature. All the brains have been affinely aligned with the Talairach standard space.

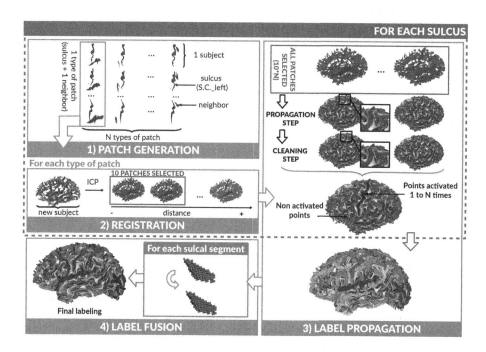

Fig. 1. Patch-based segmentation approach for automatic sulci recognition.

3.1 Patch Generation

In this paper, we experiment with a reasonable but relatively naive strategy, which will be refined in the future using machine learning. The goal is to define from the atlas dataset a library of local patches embedding enough geometrical information to minimize ambiguities when searching for a high similarity hit in the unknown subject morphology. Note that the shape of small sulci is not informative enough to prevent spurious hits. Hence the idea is to aggregate a few sulci to create discriminative local shapes. In the following, we define a type of patches for each pair of sulci that are neighbors in the brain (Fig. 1). Practically, a pair of sulci is selected if the instances of the two sulci are neighbors at least in one brain of the atlas dataset, for the topology provided by the BrainVISA pipeline yielding the folds. This pipeline endows the list of folds with a graph structure corresponding to either direct connections or to the fact that two folds are separated by a piece of gyrus. Finally, for a given sulcus S, with neighbors $S_1, S_2, ..., S_N$, N patches are generated from each atlas of the dataset, each patch corresponding to a different type of patch $SS_1, SS_2, ..., SS_N$. Note that if the neighbor or S is missing in the atlas, the patch is not included in the library.

3.2   Registration

For the registration step, the set of folds of the unknown brain and the patches of the library are represented by point clouds. The well-known iterative closest points algorithm [2] is applied to find an optimal alignment of each patch into the point cloud made up of the unlabelled folds of the unknown brain. To build the measure used to rank the matches, the nearest points in the new brain of each patch point are saved as activated points. The measure corresponds to the sum of quadratic distances of the patch points and their corresponding activated points, divided by the number of different activated points.

3.3   Label Propagation

For each patch type, the ten instances leading to the smallest distances are selected to participate to the propagation of the two parent sulci. The number of instances selected has been set to ten arbitrary for a first implementation and should be optimized later on. Note that some sulcus instances are selected several times, because they win the competition for several patch types. But their multiple contributions will be associated with slightly different alignments. Hence, sulcus instances maximizing regional similarity to the unknown subject get more weight. For each selected patch after the ICP registration to the unknown subject, each point gives its label to its nearest neighbor in the target brain. To consider the patch structure, each connected set of points in the patch should correspond to a unique connected set in the target brain: the smallest non-connected sets are excluded. Hence, each point of the target brain can be labeled several times from several patches and only the most propagated label is saved.

3.4   Label Fusion

The label fusion process is performed on a fold by fold basis. For each fold of the unknown subject, the sulcus label the most represented in its points is given to the fold. Without activated points in the fold, the "unknown" label is kept.

4 Results and Comparison with the BrainVISA Model

The proposed approach and the Bayesian BrainVISA approach are compared using a Leave-One-Out strategy on the database described above. Many different error measures are possible to evaluate the model. The measures used to evaluate the current BrainVISA model are the E_{local} for each sulcus and E_{SI} for the final

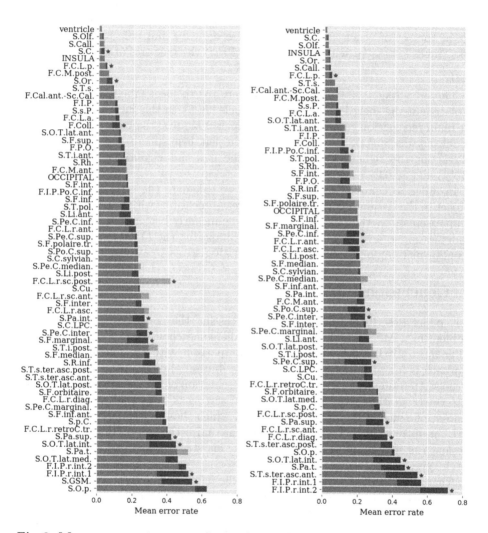

Fig. 2. Mean error rates per sulcus. The graph on the left and the graph on the right present the mean error rates for the sulci on the left hemisphere and on the right hemisphere, respectively. The Brainvisa model is represented in violet and the new model is represented in pink. The significative differences ($p_{value} < 0.05$) are marked with a star.

labeling. Here is their definitions for a given subject:

$$E_{local}(l) = \frac{FP(l) + FN(l)}{FP(l) + FN(l) + TP(l)} \; , \tag{1}$$

$$E_{SI} = \sum_{l \in L} w_l \frac{FP(l) + FN(l)}{FP(l) + FN(l) + 2TP(l)} \; , \tag{2}$$

with L the ensemble of sulcus labels, $FP(l)$, $FN(l)$ and $TP(l)$ respectively the size of the set of voxels false positive, false negative and true positive for the label l and $w_l = \frac{s_l}{\sum_{l \in L} s_l}$ with $s_l = FN(l) + TP(l)$ the true size of the sulcus with the label l.

The advantages of E_{SI} is that it is sensible to local labeling and it takes into account the shared errors between labels [9]. With this measure, we deduct the main recognition rate for the two compared models: the current BrainVISA model obtains 85.53% (+/− 5.80%) for the left hemisphere and 86.27% (+/− 6.12%) for the right hemisphere while the new model obtains 86.76% (+/− 5.16%) and 88.04% (+/− 5.70%).

In order to compare the two models, we calculate the error rates for each subject in the database and compare the set of measures with a T-test. The E_{SI} comparison shows that the new model is significantly better than the Brainvisa model ($p_{value} = 4.14e − 8$). Moreover, by comparing the E_{local} per sulcus, more than 20 sulci are found significantly better (Fig. 2).

5   Conclusion

This paper describes a first attempt at casting the cortical sulci recognition problem in a MAS-based framework. While some choices are still *ad hoc* and will require further developments, the comparison with the existing Bayesian approach is full of promise. The main contribution of our work is the extension of the MAS framework to a high level representation of the data dedicated to our pattern recognition problem. This original setting is calling for a more sophisticated inference of the library of patches, which should probably be developed with an optimization strategy trying to maximize the recognition result while keeping the library as small as possible. This strategy shall pick the selected patch types from a larger combinatorial set aggregating more than two sulci. Another improvement opportunity lies in the patch selection strategy, for example by learning the optimal cut-off for each type of patches. The label fusion could be largely improved by the introduction of weights, in order to balance the contribution of each patch according to its similarity measure. Finally, as the new strategy involves a labeling per point, it will allow the method to question the initial split of the cortex morphology into elementary folds to detect under-segmentation issues. This is an essential element to overcome the weakness of the current Bayesian framework, which is stuck to the high level representation yielded by the preprocessing stage. This possibility can be considered as a top-down feature embedded in the global recognition system.

References

1. Behnke, K.J., et al.: Automatic classification of sulcal regions of the human brain cortex using pattern recognition. In: Medical Imaging 2003: Image Processing, vol. 5032, pp. 1499–1511. International Society for Optics and Photonics (2003)
2. Besl, P.J., McKay, N.D.: Method for registration of 3-D shapes. In: Sensor Fusion IV: Control Paradigms and Data Structures, vol. 1611, pp. 586–607. International Society for Optics and Photonics (1992)
3. Blida, A.: Ontology driven graph matching approach for automatic labeling brain cortical sulci. In: IT4OD, p. 162 (2014)
4. Coupé, P., Manjón, J.V., Fonov, V., Pruessner, J., Robles, M., Collins, D.L.: Patch-based segmentation using expert priors: application to hippocampus and ventricle segmentation. NeuroImage **54**(2), 940–954 (2011)
5. Fischl, B., et al.: Automatically parcellating the human cerebral cortex. Cerebral cortex **14**(1), 11–22 (2004)
6. Jaume, S., Macq, B., Warfield, S.K.: Labeling the brain surface using a deformable multiresolution mesh. In: Dohi, T., Kikinis, R. (eds.) MICCAI 2002. LNCS, vol. 2488, pp. 451–458. Springer, Heidelberg (2002). https://doi.org/10.1007/3-540-45786-0_56
7. Lohmann, G., von Cramon, D.Y.: Automatic labelling of the human cortical surface using sulcal basins. Med. Image Anal. **4**(3), 179–188 (2000)
8. Mangin, J.F., Frouin, V., Bloch, I., Régis, J., López-Krahe, J.: From 3D magnetic resonance images to structural representations of the cortex topography using topology preserving deformations. J. Math. Imaging Vis. **5**(4), 297–318 (1995)
9. Perrot, M., Rivière, D., Mangin, J.F.: Cortical sulci recognition and spatial normalization. Med. Image Anal. **15**(4), 529–550 (2011)
10. Rivière, D., Mangin, J.F., Papadopoulos-Orfanos, D., Martinez, J.M., Frouin, V., Régis, J.: Automatic recognition of cortical sulci of the human brain using a congregation of neural networks. Med. Image Anal. **6**(2), 77–92 (2002)
11. Royackkers, N., Desvignes, M., Revenu, M.: Une méthode générale de reconnaissance de courbres 3D: application à l'identification de sillons corticaux en imagerie par résonance magnétique. Traitement du Signal **15**(5), 365–379 (1998)
12. Sandor, S., Leahy, R.: Surface-based labeling of cortical anatomy using a deformable atlas. IEEE Trans. Med. Imaging **16**(1), 41–54 (1997)
13. Shi, Y., et al.: Joint sulci detection using graphical models and boosted priors. In: Karssemeijer, N., Lelieveldt, B. (eds.) IPMI 2007. LNCS, vol. 4584, pp. 98–109. Springer, Heidelberg (2007). https://doi.org/10.1007/978-3-540-73273-0_9
14. Vivodtzev, F., Linsen, L., Hamann, B., Joy, K.I., Olshausen, B.A.: Brain mapping using topology graphs obtained by surface segmentation. In: Scientific Visualization: The Visual Extraction of Knowledge from Data, pp. 35–48. Springer, Heidelberg (2006). https://doi.org/10.1007/3-540-30790-7
15. Yang, F., Kruggel, F.: A graph matching approach for labeling brain sulci using location, orientation, and shape. Neurocomputing **73**(1–3), 179–190 (2009)

Tumor Delineation for Brain Radiosurgery by a ConvNet and Non-uniform Patch Generation

Egor Krivov[1,2]([✉]), Valery Kostjuchenko[3], Alexandra Dalechina[3],
Boris Shirokikh[1,2,4], Gleb Makarchuk[4], Alexander Denisenko[4],
Andrey Golanov[5], and Mikhail Belyaev[1,4]

[1] Kharkevich Institute for Information Transmission Problems, Moscow, Russia
e.a.krivov@gmail.com
[2] Moscow Institute of Physics and Technology, Moscow, Russia
[3] Moscow Gamma-Knife Center, Moscow, Russia
[4] Skolkovo Institute of Science and Technology, Moscow, Russia
m.belyaev@skoltech.ru
[5] Burdenko Neurosurgery Institute, Moscow, Russia

Abstract. Deep learning methods are actively used for brain lesion segmentation. One of the most popular models is DeepMedic, which was developed for segmentation of relatively large lesions like glioma and ischemic stroke. In our work, we consider segmentation of brain tumors appropriate to stereotactic radiosurgery which limits typical lesion sizes. These differences in target volumes lead to a large number of false negatives (especially for small lesions) as well as to an increased number of false positives for DeepMedic. We propose a new patch-sampling procedure to increase network performance for small lesions. We used a 6-year dataset from a stereotactic radiosurgery center. To evaluate our approach, we conducted experiments with the three most frequent brain tumors: metastasis, meningioma, schwannoma. In addition to cross-validation, we estimated quality on a hold-out test set which was collected several years later than the train one. The experimental results show solid improvements in both cases.

Keywords: Stereotactic radiosurgery · Segmentation · CNN · MRI

1 Introduction

During the last several years deep learning algorithms have gained a lot of attention from the academia since they showed previously unimaginable performance in various image analysis tasks. By now, deep learning methods are actively used in medical imaging as well [7]. In particular, deep convolutional networks dominate over traditional algorithms such as random forests in all recent MRI segmentation competitions (e.g., ischemic stroke [9] or glioma [10] segmentation).

© Springer Nature Switzerland AG 2018
W. Bai et al. (Eds.): Patch-MI 2018, LNCS 11075, pp. 122–129, 2018.
https://doi.org/10.1007/978-3-030-00500-9_14

However, we suppose that a gap exists between these results and MRI analysis in everyday clinical settings. The majority of open datasets for brain lesion segmentation are devoted to research-oriented questions such as "is it possible to extract some biomarkers associated with the clinical outcome from lesion segmentation masks?" [2]. Meanwhile, radiologists usually do not delineate lesions like glioma in their routine practice as it is a very time-consuming procedure and clinical protocols do not require it. We suppose that current deep learning-based algorithmic results lack verification in real-world clinical scenarios. Also, such verification can pose new specific requirements and therefore stimulate further algorithmic development.

In our work, we focus on adaptation of DeepMedic [6], a state-of-the-art deep learning convolutional network for brain lesion segmentation, for stereotactic radiosurgery. Delineation of pathological tissues is an obligatory part of radiosurgery planning and radiation oncologists have to detect and segment all tumors in MRI scans. So, radiosurgery is an interesting application area for deep learning methods [11]; recently two DeepMedic-based papers on brain metastasis segmentation were published [3,8]. We observe that the standard approach leads to a high number of false positives and propose a problem-oriented training procedure. To evaluate our approach, we use data on three most disseminated brain tumors (metastases, meningiomas, and acoustic schwannomas) [1] from a Gamma Knife radiosurgery center. We not only report quality metrics for cross-validation, but also provide evaluation on a test set which was collected several years later than the training one to prove robustness of the developed models. To our knowledge, it is the first time, when modern deep learning algorithms were tested over such a long period of time in the field of MRI segmentation.

2   Related Work

During the recent years, various deep learning architectures were developed. Unet, one of the most successful recent fully convolutional networks, was designed for 2D image segmentation. The core idea of the method is to add several additional connections between decoding and encoding paths to combine feature maps with various level of local and contextual information. For medical imaging, a straightforward 3D-convolutional generalization was proposed in [4]. However, a large size of typical brain MR images place some restrictions on network receptive field. In such conditions, a more simple network called DeepMedic demonstrates solid performance in series of competitions, including glioma [9] and acute ischemic stroke segmentation [10]. The network is 11 layers deep and consists of two input paths: the first process a small patch of the image in the original resolution, the second one works with larger area in a coarser resolution and provides information on patch localization. The training is based on the following patch generation algorithm: the central voxel of each patch should belong to the target mask with predefined probability.

DeepMedic was recently used in two works on brain metastases segmentation. In [8] authors modified the original architecture by adding another input branch in original resolution and reported significant improvements over the original model. Their experiments with a metastases dataset resulted in Dice score equal to 0.67. The original DeepMedic architecture was used in [3] where authors compared various combinations of T1c, T2 and Flair modalities. For T1c (in our paper we use only this modality) they reported Dice Score 0.77, sensitivity 0.92 and 10.5 false positives per image. In both papers, the original patch generation strategy was used. A non-uniform patch generation process was proposed in [5]. In fact, authors applied a predefined elastic deformation to each patch, whereas patch sampling (i.e. selection of the center voxel) was uniform.

3   Data

We focused on everyday practice of a radiosurgical center, that conducts operations with Leksell Gamma Knife. A typical Gamma Knife treatment consists of gathering patient data, frame fixation, performing an MRI scans, lesion delineation in MRI scans, treatment planning and, finally, the delivery of a dose of irradiation to a small intracranial volume through the intact skull. Delineation itself usually takes up to one hour.

We found that three of the most popular diagnoses cover 77% of all patient visits. This data is consistent with Leksell Gamma Knife society report [1], according to which in 2016 metastases, meningioma and schwannoma accounted for 70% cases treated in Gamma Knife centers. We focused only on these diagnoses since processing each new diagnosis makes our analysis more and more difficult, while clinical effect diminishes with the number of patients affected.

We use MRI T1c in all our experiments, image resolution is $(0.94, 0.94, 1)$ mm. We gathered two datasets from Gamma-Knife facility: historic and modern. Historic dataset consisted of patients examined between 2005 and 2011. Modern was gathered in 2017, we used it to ensure that developed methods could be used over a long period of time. Therefore, there was a 6 years gap between the last examination in the historic dataset and the first examination in modern dataset. Details are provided in Table 1. Ground truth was provided by medical physicists who routinely perform tumor delineation procedure.

Table 1. Total number of patients in historic and modern datasets

	Metastasis	Meningioma	Acoustic schwannoma
Historic	404	341	252
Modern	58	10	16

Metastases. Brain metastases occur when cancer cells spread from the primary tumor to the brain. Brain metastases often cause the leading clinical symptomatology in cancer, therefore their local control is very important. Survival ability of the diseased in case of applying only the supporting therapy amounts to only 40–50 days. The majority of these cases is characterized with multiple lesions, making correct tumor identification and contouring a tedious process.

Meningioma. Most meningiomas are slowly growing, benign neoplasms, deriving from arachnoid cap cells. Meningiomas are usually located on convex, cranial base, cerebral falx and tentorium. A typical meningioma is round-shaped on the side of the brain and extended on the side of the meninges. As the tumor grows, it may interfere with the normal functions of the brain. The delineation of these tumors is complicated by "dural tales" (extended part of the meninges).

Schwannoma. Vestibular schwannomas, or acoustic neuromas, are benign tumors that arise from the myelin-forming Schwann cells of the vestibulocochlear nerve. As the tumor grows, it presses hearing and vestibular fibres of the auditory nerve and the facial nerve, causing hearing loss, tinnitus (ringing in the ear) and loss of balance. If the tumor becomes larger it can affect trigeminal nerve and nearby brain structures (such as the brainstem and the cerebellum, the fourth ventricle), becoming life-threatening. A typical vestibular schwannoma looks like "comma", that arises commonly within the internal auditory meatus, and may extend into the cerebellopontine angle.

4   Method

For segmentation, we used standard DeepMedic architecture described in [6], which is also briefly described in Sect. 2.

4.1   Baseline Training Procedure

Training procedure, proposed along with DeepMedic architecture [6], consists of sampling 3D-patches from the images. Central voxels in the first half of the batch are tumorous (foreground) and are healthy (background) in the second half. Therefore, central voxels of the first half are distributed uniformly across all tumorous voxels. This sampling procedure is used to fight class imbalance, since foreground voxels are much rarer than background voxels.

4.2   Tumor Sampling (TS)

After training our baseline model we discovered that sensitivity was relatively low both in test and train sets. We concluded that the model was not trained well enough. Having observed false negative cases in the training set, we found that many of them were small metastases in a brain which had both big (Fig. 1) and small (Fig. 2) metastases. Original sampling procedure would strongly favour sampling from big metastasis in this case, significantly decreasing number of small metastases observed during training. To fix that we change foreground sampling procedure. Instead of uniformly choosing foreground voxels we first randomly choose a metastasis and only then pick a random voxel inside. This means that now all metastases are equally represented in training set, including the smallest ones.

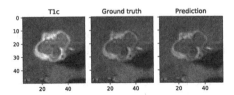

Fig. 1. TP prediction of easy-to-detect tumor

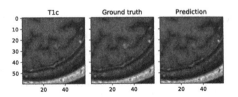

Fig. 2. FN prediction of the small tumor

4.3   High Intensity Sampling (HIS)

Observing false positive cases we found out that there are many of false predictions in the structures with high intensity level (Fig. 3) and in some parts of skull. To prevent our model from making such prediction and also to improve predictions near high intensity structures (Fig. 4), we change sampling procedure almost the same way. Voxels with more than 90-th percentile intensity were chosen as High Intensity class. Then, instead of uniformly choosing a background voxel, we firstly made a decision between High Intensity class (with probability 0.3) and standard sampling procedure from the background. This approach allows algorithm to learn from hard-to-recognize structures more often.

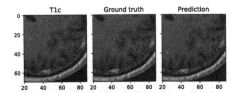

Fig. 3. FP prediction of high intensity structures

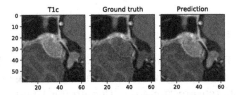

Fig. 4. FN predictions of near high intensity structures

5   Experiments

Measuring Performance. The tumor delineation process could be considered a tumor detection followed by its segmentation. Detection is a process of spotting the tumors; segmentation is the process of contouring these tumors close to the way the physician did. Detection quality can be measured by using sensitivity and number of false positives computed for tumors. Here we define that tumor was found if there was an intersection between predicted tumor and true tumor. Segmentation quality can be measured by Dice similarity coefficient computed for all patient's voxels. It's a popular metric widely used in segmentation tasks.

Training Procedure Parameters. During our preliminary experiments we discovered that sampling foreground voxel with probability 0.5 lead to the large number of false positive examples, so we decreased this probability to 0.25. During training we are using patch size of 15 as an output of our model, since this increases sensitivity and dice score in our case. We train our models for 120 epochs since training loss plateaus at this point for any learning rate. Each epoch consists of 200 stochastic gradient descent iterations. We start our training with learning rate of 0.1, and halve it whenever training loss plateaus.

Data Preprocessing. We didn't use standard preprocessing techniques like brain extraction since it can take dozens of minutes. In clinical settings it could annihilate all acceleration of delineation process obtained by deep learning.

Reproducibility. We conducted our experiments using Python and PyTorch. Our deep learning algorithms are written in a highly modular way and fully reproducible thanks to usage of Docker containers. We haven't released it at the moment to preserve anonymity during double-blind reviewing.

5.1   Results for Cross-Validation

First we evaluate our algorithms on each dataset with 5-fold cross validation. Results are presented in Table 2. We do not apply Tumor Sampling for schwannoma segmentation since most of the corresponding patients have only one tumor.

Table 2. Results of a 5-fold cross-validation on the historic dataset, TS - Tumor Sampling, HIS - High Intensity Sampling.

Setting	Metastasis			Meningioma			Schwannoma		
	Dice	Sensitivity	FP	Dice	Sensitivity	FP	Dice	Sensitivity	FP
Baseline	0.787	0.898	8.3	0.735	0.929	6.9	0.881	0.975	1.6
TS	0.792	0.932	6.6	0.737	0.933	5.6	-	-	-
HIS	0.791	0.904	7.5	0.731	0.925	4.9	0.874	0.979	1.7
TS & HIS	0.798	0.946	11.8	0.742	0.928	4.6	-	-	-

5.2   Testing on Modern Data

After that we retrain our algorithm on each historic dataset (2006–2011) and test them on modern dataset, which was gathered six years later (2017). Results are presented in Table 3, see also Fig. 5 for examples of predicted masks. For meningioma segmentation HIS showed significant increase in dice score. We checked results more precisely: methods differed in how they predicted tumor attached to the skull, with HIS being much more accurate.

These results demonstrates that our algorithm is quite robust to the typical changes of this center, since if we had been able to provide our algorithm six years

Table 3. Experiments on different tumors, TS - Tumor Sampling, HIS - High Intensity Sampling. We used the historic dataset (2006–2011) for training and the modern one (2017) as a hold-out test set to calculate quality metrics

	Metastasis			Meningioma			Schwannoma		
Setting	Dice	Sensitivity	FP	Dice	Sensitivity	FP	Dice	Sensitivity	FP
Baseline	0.807	0.856	7.4	0.615	0.927	4.3	0.793	0.962	1.8
TS	0.799	0.912	5.2	0.604	0.927	3.4	-	-	-
HIS	0.799	0.849	5.0	0.697	0.927	2.5	0.8	0.962	1.4
TS & HIS	0.789	0.911	4.7	0.685	0.936	2.4	-	-	-

ago, it would still provide reasonable quality up until this moment. Also, since we could use different algorithms for detection and segmentation, we could always have the best of different models, combining best dice score and sensitivity/FP.

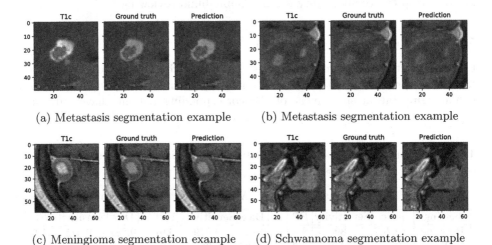

(a) Metastasis segmentation example   (b) Metastasis segmentation example

(c) Meningioma segmentation example   (d) Schwannoma segmentation example

Fig. 5. Examples of predicted masks for Tumor Sampling method. Each subfigure contains a T1c image (left), expert annotation (center) and prediction (right)

6   Conclusion

We developed a new patch sampling strategy to meet needs of delineating brain lesions for radiosurgery and evaluated the proposed approach by segmenting three of the most common tumors. Also, we emulate long-term usage of our deep learning-based system in clinical settings and demonstrated robust performance of the method.

Acknowledgements. The results of sections 1, 2, 4 and 5 are based on the scientific research conducted at IITP RAS and supported by the Russian Science Foundation under grant 17-11-01390.

References

1. Leksell gamma knife society: patients treated with leksell gamma knife 1968–2016. https://www.lgksociety.com/library/annual-treatment-statistics/
2. Bakas, S., et al.: Advancing the cancer genome atlas glioma MRI collections with expert segmentation labels and radiomic features (2017)
3. Charron, O., Lallement, A., Jarnet, D., Noblet, V., Clavier, J.B., Meyer, P.: Automatic detection and segmentation of brain metastases on multimodal MR images with a deep convolutional neural network. Comput. Biol. Med. **95**, 43–54 (2018)
4. Çiçek, Ö., Abdulkadir, A., Lienkamp, S.S., Brox, T., Ronneberger, O.: 3D U-Net: learning dense volumetric segmentation from sparse annotation. In: Ourselin, S., Joskowicz, L., Sabuncu, M.R., Unal, G., Wells, W. (eds.) MICCAI 2016. LNCS, vol. 9901, pp. 424–432. Springer, Cham (2016). https://doi.org/10.1007/978-3-319-46723-8_49
5. Ghafoorian, M., et al.: Non-uniform patch sampling with deep convolutional neural networks for white matter hyperintensity segmentation. In: 2016 IEEE 13th International Symposium on Biomedical Imaging (ISBI), pp. 1414–1417. IEEE (2016)
6. Kamnitsas, K., et al.: Efficient multi-scale 3D CNN with fully connected crf for accurate brain lesion segmentation. Med. Image Anal. **36**, 61–78 (2017)
7. Litjens, G., et al.: A survey on deep learning in medical image analysis. Med. Image Anal. **42**, 60–88 (2017)
8. Liu, Y., et al.: A deep convolutional neural network-based automatic delineation strategy for multiple brain metastases stereotactic radiosurgery. PloS ONE **12**(10), e0185844 (2017)
9. Maier, O., et al.: ISLES 2015-A public evaluation benchmark for ischemic stroke lesion segmentation from multispectral MRI. Med. Image Anal. **35**, 250–269 (2017)
10. Menze, B.H., et al.: The multimodal brain tumor image segmentation benchmark (BRATS). IEEE Trans. Med. Imaging **34**(10), 1993–2024 (2015)
11. Zaharchuk, G., Gong, E., Wintermark, M., Rubin, D., Langlotz, C.: Deep learning in neuroradiology. Am. J. Neuroradiol. (2018)

Retinal Image Analysis

Iterative Deep Retinal Topology Extraction

Carles Ventura[1]([✉]), Jordi Pont-Tuset[2], Sergi Caelles[2], Kevis-Kokitsi Maninis[2], and Luc Van Gool[2]

[1] Scene Understading and Artificial Intelligence Lab, Universitat Oberta de Catalunya, Barcelona, Spain
cventuraroy@uoc.edu
[2] Computer Vision Laboratory ETH Zürich, Zürich, Switzerland
{jponttuset,scaelles,kmaninis,vangool}@vision.ee.ethz.ch

Abstract. This paper tackles the task of estimating the topology of filamentary networks such as retinal vessels. Building on top of a global model that performs a dense semantical classification of the pixels of the image, we design a Convolutional Neural Network (CNN) that predicts the local connectivity between the central pixel of an input patch and its border points. By iterating this local connectivity we sweep the whole image and infer the global topology of the filamentary network, inspired by a human delineating a complex network with the tip of their finger. We perform a qualitative and quantitative evaluation on retinal veins and arteries topology extraction on DRIVE dataset, where we show superior performance to very strong baselines.

1 Introduction

Deep learning has gone a long way since its jump to fame in the field of computer vision thanks to the outstanding results in the Imagenet [23] image classification competition back in 2012 [11]. We have witnessed the appearance of deeper [24] and deeper [10] architectures and the generalization to object detection [6,7, 21]. Convolutional Neural Networks (CNNs) have played a central role in this development.

A significant step forward was done with the introduction of CNNs for dense prediction, in which the output of the system was not a classification of an image or bounding box into certain categories, but each pixel would receive an output decision. Many tasks have been tackled from this perspective since then: semantic instance segmentation [9,14], edge detection [29], medical image segmentation [15], etc.

Other tasks, however, have a richer output structure beyond a per-pixel classification, and a higher abstraction of the result is expected. Notable examples that have already been tackled by CNNs are the estimation of the human pose [19], or the room layout [13] from an image. The common denominator of these tasks is that one expects an abstracted model of the result rather than a set of pixel classifications.

© Springer Nature Switzerland AG 2018
W. Bai et al. (Eds.): Patch-MI 2018, LNCS 11075, pp. 133–143, 2018.
https://doi.org/10.1007/978-3-030-00500-9_15

This work falls into this category by bringing the power of CNNs to the estimation of the **topology of filamentary networks** such as retinal vessels. The structured output is of critical importance and priceless value in these applications: rather than knowing exactly which pixels in a retinal image are vessels or not, detecting whether two points are connected and how is arguably more informative.

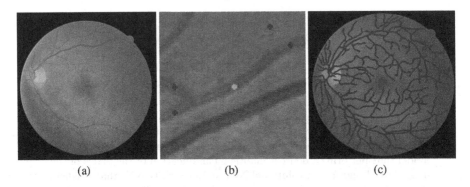

(a)   (b)   (c)

Fig. 1. Patch-based iterative approach for network topology extraction. (a): Input retinal image. (b): detections at the local patch for the points at the border (in green) connected to the central point (in blue). (c): final result once the iterative approach ends. (Color figure online)

If one thinks how humans would extract the topology of an entangled graph network from an image, it might quickly come to mind the image of them tracing the filaments with the finger and *sweeping* the connected paths continuously. Inspired by this, we propose an iterative deep learning approach that sequentially connects dots within the filaments until it *sweeps* all the visible network. Our approach naturally allows incorporating human corrections: one can simply restart the tracing from the corrected point.

Tracing of curvilinear structures has been of broad interest in a range of applications, varying from blood vessel segmentation, roadmap segmentation, and reconstruction of human vasculature. Hessian-based methods rely on derivatives, to guide the development of a snake [28], or to detect vessel boundaries [1]. Model-based methods rely on strong assumptions about the geometric shapes of the filamentary structures [12,26]. Learning-based methods emerged for the task, using SVMs on line operators [22], fully-connected CRFs [20], gradient-boosting [2], classification trees [8], or nearest neighbours [25]. Closer to our approach, the most recent methods rely on Fully Convolutional Neural Networks (FCNs), to segment retinal blood vessels [5,15], or recover vascular boundaries [18]. Different than all the aforementioned method that result in binary structure maps, our method employs deep learning to trace the entire structure of the curvilinear structures, recovering their entire connectivity map.

More specifically, we train a CNN on small patches that localizes input and output points of the filaments within the patch (Fig. 1(b)). By iteratively connecting these dots we obtain the global topology (graph) of the network (Fig. 1(c)). We tackle the extraction of the topology of retinal vessels (veins and arteries) from fundus images. We experiment on DRIVE dataset to show that our algorithm improves over some very strong baselines and provides accurate representations of the topology of vessels. To the best of our knowledge, we are the first to apply deep learning for tracing curvilinear structures. Code is available in https://github.com/carlesventura/iterative-deep-retinal.

2   Our Approach

This section presents our approach, which combines a global scale for curvilinear structure segmentation and a local scale to estimate its connectivity. The current best approaches for curvilinear structure segmentation applies state-of-the-art deep learning techniques to obtain a segmentation map where each pixel is classified as belonging to the structure (foreground) or not (background). The most relevant example of such approach is the VGG-based architecture used in DRIU [15] for vessel segmentation. Despite their good performance in segmentation evaluation measures, one of the main drawbacks of these approaches is that they do not take any structure information into account. In particular, this method is blind to connectivity information among the points that lie in their predicted mask, since all points are assigned only a binary label.

Section 2.1 proposes a method that learns the connectivity of the elements at a local scale. Once the local model is learned, it is iteratively applied to the image, connecting previous predictions with next ones, and gradually extracting the topology of the network, as explained in Sect. 2.2. The evaluation metrics are presented in Sect. 2.3.

2.1   Patch-Level Learning for Connectivity

As introduced above, the goal is to train a model to estimate the local connectivity in patches. The concept of connectivity is not a property from single points but from pairs of pixels. Current architectures, however, are designed to estimate per-pixel properties rather than pairwise information. To solve this issue, the local network is designed to estimate which points in a patch are connected to a given input point.

More precisely, we take the architecture of stacked hourglass networks [19] to learn the patch-based model for connectivity. This architecture is based on a repeated bottom-up, top-down processing used in conjunction with intermediate supervision. Each bottom-up, top-down processing block is referred to as an hourglass module, which is related to fully convolutional networks that process spatial information at multiple scales but with a more symmetric distribution.

The network is trained using a set of $k \times k$-pixel patches from the training set with the pixel at the center of the patch belonging to the foreground (e.g. a vessel). The output is a heatmap that predicts the probability of each location being connected to the central point of the patch.

Furthermore, the model is also trained to differentiate between the two types of vessel (arteries or veins), so the model is forced to learn not only the connectivity but also an artery-vein classification problem. To illustrate this idea, Fig. 2 shows some examples of connectivity for retinal images where we differentiate three types of models. Figures 2(a) and (b) compare two patches where all vessels that intersect the border patch have been marked (Fig. 2(a)), versus the ones that are connected to the vessel at the center of the patch (Fig. 2(b)). Figures 2(c) and (d) illustrate the difference between detecting the connectivity over any type of vessel (Fig. 2(c)), or forcing the connectivity to be over the same type of vessel (Fig. 2(d)).

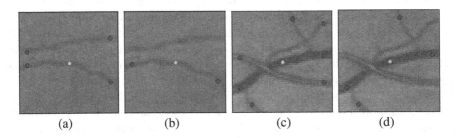

(a)	(b)	(c)	(d)

Fig. 2. Examples of training patches for connectivity. The green points represent the locations from the patch border connected with the vessel indicated by the blue point in the center. (Color figure online)

We finally connect the border locations to the center locations by computing the shortest path through the semantic segmentation computed from the global model introduced before. Note that the patch is local enough that a shortest path on the global model is reliable.

2.2   Iterative Delineation

Once the patch-level model for connectivity has been learned, the model is applied iteratively through the image in order to extract the topology of the network. We start from the point with highest foreground probability, given by the global model. We then center a patch on this point and find the set of locations at the border of the patch that are connected to the center using the local patch model.

We discard the locations with a confidence value below a certain threshold and add the remaining ones to a bag of points to be explored B_E. For each predicted point, we store its location, its confidence value and its precedent predicted point (i.e. the point that was on the center of the patch when the point was predicted). The predicted point p from B_E with the highest confidence value is removed from B_E and inserted to a list of visited points B_V. Then, p is connected to its precedent predicted point using the Dijkstra [3] algorithm over the segmentation probability map over the patch to find the minimum path between them.

We then iterate the process with a patch centered on p_c and the new predicted points over the confidence threshold are appended to B_E where they will *compete* against the previous points in B_E to be the next point to be explored. This process is iteratively applied until B_E is empty. Note that the list of visited points B_V is used to discard any point already explored and, therefore, to avoid revisiting the same points. In a patch centered on p_c, if a predicted point p_p belongs to a local neighbourhood of a point $p_v \in B_V$ and p_v is the precedent point of p_c, then the predicted point p_p is discarded. Otherwise, if p_v is not the precedent point of p_c but p_p belongs to a local neighbourhood of p_v, then the predicted point p_p is considered to be connected with p_c, but p_p will not be considered for expansion.

Since in retinal images all vessels are connected through the optical disk, any vessel point from the image is reachable from any starting point used in the iterative approach. However, the algorithm has been generalized to tackle a problem with unconnected areas, e.g. a cropped retinal image where the entire retina is not visible and, therefore, there could be vessels not reachable from a single starting point. To prevent that some part of the network topology may have not been extracted, we select a new starting point for a new exploration once the previous B_E is empty. We impose two constraints on the eligibility for a new starting point: (*i*) they have to be at a minimum distance of the areas already explored and (*ii*) their confidence value on the segmentation probability map has to be over a minimum confidence threshold.

2.3   Topology Evaluation

The output of our algorithm is a graph defining the topology of the input network, so we need metrics to evaluate their correctness. We propose two different measures for this: a *classical* precision-recall measure that evaluates which locations of the network are detected, and a metric to evaluate connectivity, by quantifying how many pairs of points are correctly or incorrectly connected.

To compute the classical precision-recall curve between two graphs, we build an image with a pixel-wide line sweeping all edges of the given graphs. We then apply the original precision-recall for boundaries [16] on these pair of images. Precision P refers to the ratio between the number of pixels correctly detected as boundary (true positives) and the number of pixels detected as boundary (true positives + false positives). Recall R refers to the ratio between the number of pixels correctly detected as boundary (true positives) and the number of pixels annotated as boundary in the ground truth (true positive + false negative). We take the F measure between P and R as a trade-off metric.

The second measure is the connectivity C, inspired by the definition in [17] as the ratio of segments which were estimated without discontinuities. We define a segment in the graph as the curvilinear structure that connects two consecutive junctions in the ground-truth annotations, as well as connecting an endpoint and its closest connected junction (junctions refer to both crossovers and bifurcations). Two junctions are considered consecutive if there is no other junction within the line that connects them. Given the ground truth path between two consecutive junctions p_{gt}, the nearest point from the predicted network to each junction is retrieved. Then, the shortest path through the predicted network connecting the retrieved pair of points is computed, which is referred to as p_{pred}. If the ratio between the length of p_{gt} and the length of p_{pred} is greater than 0.8 we consider that the ground truth path p_{gt} has been estimated without discontinuities. In Fig. 3, the two images on the left show examples where the ground truth segment have been estimated without discontinuities, whereas the two examples on the right are considered as not connected segments on the connectivity measure.

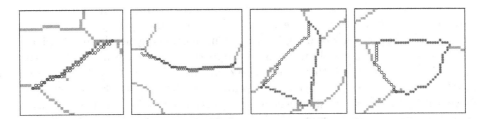

Fig. 3. Examples of good (on the left) and bad (on the right) connectivity. Green pixels represent ground truth connections, blue pixels represent predicted vessels with our iterative approach and red pixels represent the path found through predicted network. (Color figure online)

We propose to also have an F measure that combines precision P with connectivity C. The reason is that a high connectivity C value does not implies a good graph that defines the topology of the network. Whereas the connectivity measures the ratio of estimated segments without discontinuities, the precision measures how good the predicted locations along the segments are. For the rest of the paper, F^R stands for the F measure computed with recall and precision for boundaries values, whereas F^C stands for the F measure computed between connectivity and precision.

3   Experiments

The experiments have been carried out on the DRIVE [27] dataset, which includes 40 eye fundus images and contains manual segmentation of the blood vessels by expert annotators. As a global model for segmentation, we use DRIU [15], which is the state of the art for retinal vessel segmentation.

Patch-level evaluation: To train the patch-level model for connectivity we randomly select 50 patches with size 64 × 64 pixels from each image of the training set, all of them centered on one of vertices of the graph annotations provided by [4], which includes arteries and veins annotations. The ground-truth locations for the connectivity at the patch level are found by intersecting the vessels with a square of side s pixels (slightly smaller than the patch size) centered on the patch. The ground-truth output heatmap is then generated by adding some Gaussian peaks centered in a subset of the found locations, depending on the configuration:

- For the *non-connectivity* model, all the locations are considered (Fig. 2(a)).
- For the *connectivity* model, only the intersection points connected to the center along a path completely included in the patch are considered (Figs. 2(b) and (c)).
- For the *connectivity-av* model, only the intersection points connected to the center and belonging to the same type of vessel (artery or vein) as the vessel centered on the patch are considered (Fig. 2(d)).

The non-connectivity patch-level model reaches the best result (F = 82.1, P = 85.3, R = 79.1). The connectivity model, which has to tell apart those points connected with the patch center, achieves an only slightly worse performance (F = 80.4, P = 82.5, R = 78.4), despite the task being more complicated. The model that has also to distinguish between arteries and veins results in a more significant drop in the performance (F = 74.8, P = 75.9, R = 73.7), but it still keeps a very good result.

Figure 4 shows some visual results for the three type of configurations considered. In the first row, the model is able to differentiate the vessels connected to the patch center from those ones not connected (3rd and 4th column). In the second row, the model differentiates the vessels from the same type as the centered vessel (an artery) from those of different vessel type (see 4th and 5th column). The last row shows a failure case where the model correctly predicts the connectivity but it is not able to differentiate the arteries from the veins.

Iterative delineation: Once the patch-level model for connectivity has been trained, it is iteratively applied to extract the topology of the blood vessels networks from the eye fundus images. As a strong baseline we compare to extracting the morphological skeleton of detections binarized at different thresholds from the architecture proposed in DRIU [15], a VGG base network on which a set of specialized layers are trained to solve the retinal vessel segmentation task. Our proposed iterative approach uses this VGG-based architecture as the global model to select the starting point and to connect the points detected by the patch-level model with the central point of the patch (see Sect. 2.2). Table 1 compares to DRIU for different thresholds: 224 (the optimal for vessel segmentation obtained in [15]), 200 (the optimal value for precision-recall boundary evaluation F^R) and 170 (the optimal value for precision-connectivity evaluation F^C). Our proposed iterative approach outperforms DRIU for connectivity in 6.6 points, which results on a improvement of 1.8 in the precision-connectivity evaluation measure F^C. Furthermore, both techniques are also compared with an upper bound and a lower bound: the former is the skeleton extracted from the ground truth vessel segmentation, and the latter results from evaluating the

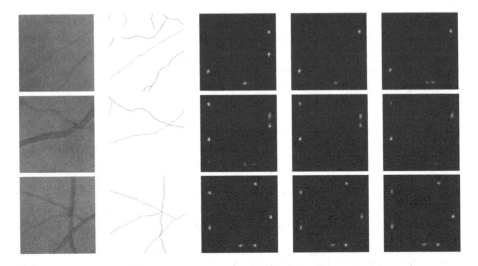

Fig. 4. Visual results of the patch-level models for eye fundus images. From left to right: eye fundus image, artery-vein annotation, output confidence for non-connectivity model, output confidence for connectivity model and output confidence for connectivity-av (artery-vein) model.

ground truth skeleton obtained from a different image. Our results are only 7.7 points below the upper bound in connectivity. The experiments have also been performed with other patch size values ($k = 32$ and $k = 128$) and the results do not change significantly, which shows the robustness of the patch size to the scale of the image. PSPNet [30], which is the state-of-the-art semantic segmentation method to date, has also been considered as a baseline. However, the results obtained by PSPNet in the DRIVE dataset are significanlty lower compared to DRIU [15] (see Table 1).

Figure 5 illustrates how the vessel network topology extraction evolves along the iterations of our proposed approach for one of the test images.

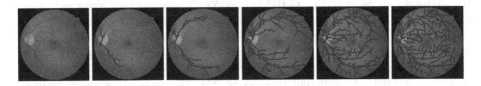

Fig. 5. Evolution of the vessel network in the iterative delineation.

Arteries and veins separation: For eye fundus images, we also pursue the objective of differentiating arteries and veins. The approach is similar to the iterative delineation proposed before, but now using the patch-level model for connectivity that also takes into account that the vessels connected have to be of the same type. We have referred before to this model as the *connectivity-av* model.

Table 1. Boundary Precision-Recall and Connectivity evaluation for vessels (left), arteries (top-right) and veins (bottom-right) in the DRIVE dataset

	P	R	C	F^R	F^C
DRIU-224 [15]	**97.3**	84.7	67.7	90.4	79.8
DRIU-200 [15]	93.8	90.6	74.0	**92.0**	82.7
DRIU-170 [15]	89.9	93.1	78.3	91.3	83.7
PSPNet [30]	92.8	69.9	49.7	79.5	64.7
Iterative (ours)	86.1	**94.1**	**84.9**	89.8	**85.5**
GT skel (upperbound)	95.6	99.3	92.6	97.4	94.1
Random (lowerbound)	44.2	45.9	21.8	44.9	29.2

	P	R	C	F^R	F^C
VGG-220	72.9	80.7	52.4	76.1	61.0
VGG-190	64.5	**88.2**	**65.4**	74.1	64.9
Iterative (ours)	**81.4**	75.3	63.0	**78.0**	**71.0**
VGG-230	70.8	79.1	42.2	74.2	52.9
VGG-180	57.4	**91.3**	**66.1**	70.2	61.5
Iterative (ours)	**72.0**	79.6	61.2	**75.4**	**66.2**

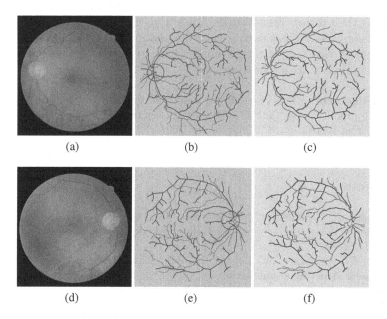

(a)   (b)   (c)

(d)   (e)   (f)

Fig. 6. Qualitative results on arteries and veins separation for two test images ((a) and (d)) comparing ground truth ((b) and (e)) with our method ((c) and (f)): veins in blue, arteries in red. (Color figure online)

As baseline, we have considered the same CNN architecture as in DRIU, i.e. a VGG-based architecture, but using the annotations for arteries and veins given by [4]. These annotations are only given at the graph level, so we build the ground-truth image by drawing one-pixel wide lines delineating the arteries and veins networks; which is different from the vessel segmentation pixel-accurate masks from DRIVE on which DRIU is usually trained. We train one global model for arteries and one for veins, and then we apply the delineation algorithm using the connectivity-av patch-level model. Table 1 shows the results obtained for arteries (top-right) and veins (bottom-right). In both cases, our iterative approach reaches the best trade off between F^R and F^C. Figure 6 shows some qualitative results comparing the ground truth annotations with our method.

4   Conclusions

In this paper we have presented an approach that iteratively applies a patch-based CNN model for connectivity to extract the topology of filamentary networks. We have demonstrated the effectiveness of our technique on retinal vessels from fundus images. The patch-based model is capable of learning that the central point is the input location and of finding the locations at the patch border connected to the center. Furthermore, we can also differentiate arteries and veins and extract their respective networks. A new F measure (F^C) that combines precision and connectivity has been proposed to evaluate the topology results. The experiments carried out on retinal images have obtained the best performance on F^C compared to strong baselines.

Acknowledgements. This research was supported by the Spanish Ministry of Economy and Competitiveness (TIN2015-66951-C2-2-R grant), by Swiss Commission for Technology and Innovation (CTI, Grant No. 19015.1 PFES-ES, NeGeVA) and by the Universitat Oberta de Catalunya.

References

1. Bankhead, P., Scholfield, C.N., McGeown, J.G., Curtis, T.M.: Fast retinal vessel detection and measurement using wavelets and edge location refinement. PloS one **7**, e32435 (2012)
2. Becker, C., Rigamonti, R., Lepetit, V., Fua, P.: Supervised feature learning for curvilinear structure segmentation. In: MICCAI (2013)
3. Dijkstra, E.: A note on two problems in connexion with graphs. Numerische Mathematik **1**, (1959)
4. Estrada, R., Allingham, M.J., Mettu, P.S., Cousins, S.W., Tomasi, C., Farsiu, S.: Retinal artery-vein classification via topology estimation. T-MI **34**, (2015)
5. Fu, H., Xu, Y., Lin, S., Kee Wong, D.W., Liu, J.: DeepVessel: retinal vessel segmentation via deep learning and conditional random field. In: Ourselin, S., Joskowicz, L., Sabuncu, M.R., Unal, G., Wells, W. (eds.) MICCAI 2016. LNCS, vol. 9901, pp. 132–139. Springer, Cham (2016). https://doi.org/10.1007/978-3-319-46723-8_16
6. Girshick, R.: Fast R-CNN. In: ICCV (2015)
7. Girshick, R., Donahue, J., Darrell, T., Malik, J.: Rich feature hierarchies for accurate object detection and semantic segmentation. In: CVPR (2014)
8. Gu, L., Cheng, L.: Learning to boost filamentary structure segmentation. In: ICCV (2015)
9. He, K., Gkioxari, G., Dollár, P., Girshick, R.: Mask R-CNN. In: ICCV (2017)
10. He, K., Zhang, X., Ren, S., Sun, J.: Deep residual learning for image recognition. In: CVPR (2016)
11. Krizhevsky, A., Sutskever, I., Hinton, G.E.: Imagenet classification with deep convolutional neural networks. In: NIPS (2012)

12. Law, M.W.K., Chung, A.C.S.: Three dimensional curvilinear structure detection using optimally oriented flux. In: Forsyth, D., Torr, P., Zisserman, A. (eds.) ECCV 2008. LNCS, vol. 5305, pp. 368–382. Springer, Heidelberg (2008). https://doi.org/10.1007/978-3-540-88693-8_27

13. Lee, C.Y., Badrinarayanan, V., Malisiewicz, T., Rabinovich, A.: Roomnet: End-to-end room layout estimation. In: ICCV (2017)

14. Li, Y., Qi, H., Dai, J., Ji, X., Wei, Y.: Fully convolutional instance-aware semantic segmentation. In: CVPR (2017)

15. Maninis, K.-K., Pont-Tuset, J., Arbeláez, P., Van Gool, L.: Deep retinal image understanding. In: Ourselin, S., Joskowicz, L., Sabuncu, M.R., Unal, G., Wells, W. (eds.) MICCAI 2016. LNCS, vol. 9901, pp. 140–148. Springer, Cham (2016). https://doi.org/10.1007/978-3-319-46723-8_17

16. Martin, D.R., Fowlkes, C.C., Malik, J.: Learning to detect natural image boundaries using local brightness, color, and texture cues. In: TPAMI (2004)

17. Máttyus, G., Luo, W., Urtasun, R.: Deeproadmapper: Extracting road topology from aerial images. In: International Conference on Computer Vision (2017)

18. Merkow, J., Marsden, A., Kriegman, D., Tu, Z.: Dense volume-to-volume vascular boundary detection. In: Ourselin, S., Joskowicz, L., Sabuncu, M.R., Unal, G., Wells, W. (eds.) MICCAI 2016. LNCS, vol. 9902, pp. 371–379. Springer, Cham (2016). https://doi.org/10.1007/978-3-319-46726-9_43

19. Newell, A., Yang, K., Deng, J.: Stacked hourglass networks for human pose estimation. In: Leibe, B., Matas, J., Sebe, N., Welling, M. (eds.) ECCV 2016. LNCS, vol. 9912, pp. 483–499. Springer, Cham (2016). https://doi.org/10.1007/978-3-319-46484-8_29

20. Orlando, J.I., Blaschko, M.: Learning fully-connected CRFs for blood vessel segmentation in retinal images. In: Golland, P., Hata, N., Barillot, C., Hornegger, J., Howe, R. (eds.) MICCAI 2014. LNCS, vol. 8673, pp. 634–641. Springer, Cham (2014). https://doi.org/10.1007/978-3-319-10404-1_79

21. Ren, S., He, K., Girshick, R., Sun, J.: Faster R-CNN: Towards real-time object detection with region proposal networks. In: NIPS (2015)

22. Ricci, E., Perfetti, R.: Retinal blood vessel segmentation using line operators and support vector classification. T-MI **26**, (2007)

23. Russakovsky, O.: ImageNet large scale visual recognition challenge. IJCV **115**, 211–252 (2015)

24. Simonyan, K., Zisserman, A.: Very deep convolutional networks for large-scale image recognition. In: ICLR (2015)

25. Sironi, A., Lepetit, V., Fua, P.: Projection onto the manifold of elongated structures for accurate extraction. In: ICCV (2015)

26. Soares, J.V., Leandro, J.J., Cesar Jr, R.M., Jelinek, H.F., Cree, M.J.: Retinal vessel segmentation using the 2-D gabor wavelet and supervised classification. T-MI **25**, (2006)

27. Staal, J., Abramoff, M., Niemeijer, M., Viergever, M., van Ginneken, B.: Ridge based vessel segmentation in color images of the retina. T-MI **23**, (2004)

28. Wang, Y., Narayanaswamy, A., Tsai, C.L., Roysam, B.: A broadly applicable 3-D neuron tracing method based on open-curve snake. Neuroinformatics **9**, 193–217 (2011)

29. Xie, S., Tu, Z.: Holistically-nested edge detection. IJCV **125**, (2017)

30. Zhao, H., Shi, J., Qi, X., Wang, X., Jia, J.: Pyramid scene parsing network. In: CVPR (2017)

Author Index

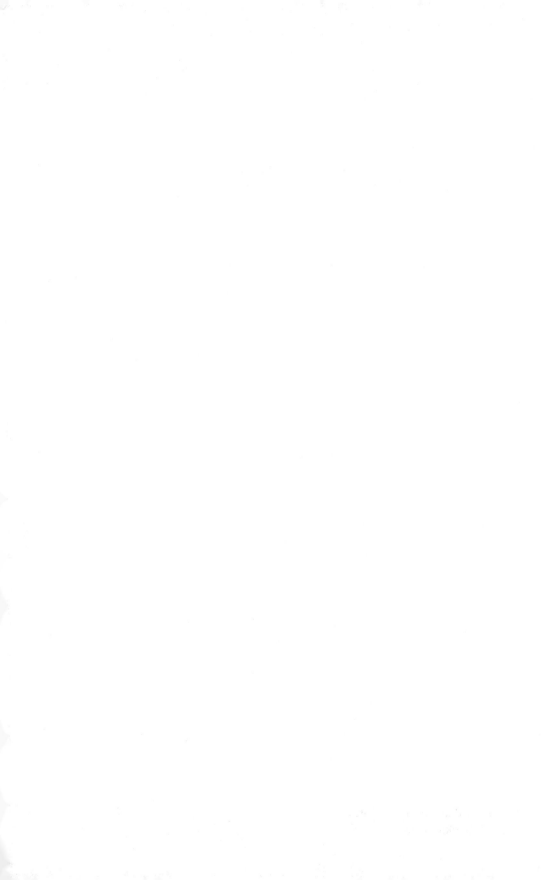

Printed in the United States
By Bookmasters